365 WODs

BURPEES, DEADLIFTS, SNATCHES, SQUATS,
BOX JUMPS, SITUPS, KETTLEBELL SWINGS,
DOUBLE UNDERS, LUNGES, PUSHUPS, PULLUPS, AND
MORE DAILY WORKOUTS FOR HOME, AT THE GYM,
AND ON THE ROAD

Blair Morrison, personal trainer and CrossFit Games® finalist

Fair Winds Press
100 Cummings Center, Suite 406L
Beverly, MA 01915

fairwindspress.com • bodymindbeautyhealth.com

First published in the USA in 2015 by
Fair Winds Press, a member of
Quarto Publishing Group USA Inc.
100 Cummings Center
Suite 406-L
Beverly, MA 01915-6101
www.fairwindspress.com
Visit www.bodymindbeautyhealth.com. It's your personal guide to a happy, healthy, and extraordinary life!

19 18 17 16 15   1 2 3 4 5

ISBN: 978-1-59233-637-1

Digital edition published in 2015
eISBN: 978-1-62788-278-1
Library of Congress Cataloging-in-Publication Data available

Cover design by Mattie Wells
Book design by Mattie Wells
Photography by Shelly Hull; except where noted

Printed and bound in China

The information in this book is for educational purposes only. It is not intended to replace the advice of a physician or medical practitioner. Please see your health care provider before beginning any new health program.

CONTENTS

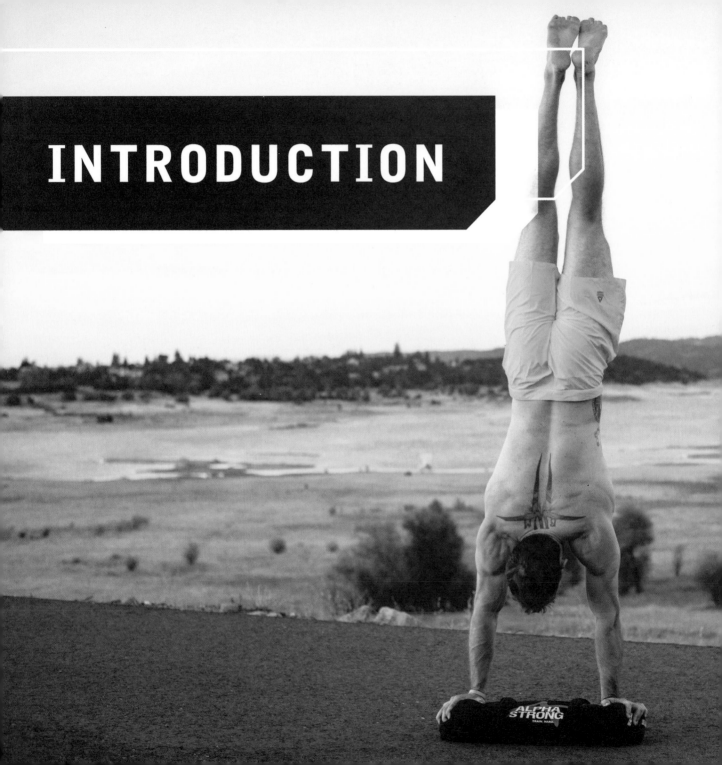

INTRODUCTION

WHAT IS A WOD?

A **WOD** is the workout of the day. The goal of a properly organized training program is to constantly vary these workouts by movement type, duration, and combination. This ensures the body will never slip into a routine and eliminate the stimulus to improve. By choosing only from exercises that are "functional" (movements that are naturally occurring during our daily lives), a good program provides its participants with general physical preparedness for any challenge they might face. For example, a squat allows us to practice the movement of sitting down and standing up. A deadlift allows us to practice lifting something off the ground. Finally, by performing these varied movements at high intensity, we are able to challenge not only the muscles but the heart and lungs as well. The idea that "cardio" needs to be an hour on the treadmill no longer applies.

WHO IS THIS FOR?

This book is for the traditional gym-goer looking for a new twist on fitness, the budding fitness enthusiast needing resources on how to balance training, or the fitness minimalist who enjoys creating a workout with as little equipment as possible. The movements and exercises included are intended to be easily adapted to a range of environments and fitness situations; therefore, you will not be required to go out and buy a bunch of equipment or sign up for an expensive gym membership in order to follow this program. If you already have a membership to a gym, *365 WODs* will make that experience only more enjoyable and productive.

WHAT LEVEL OF FITNESS IS REQUIRED?

365 WODs is designed to be adaptable for the vast majority of fitness levels. Barring serious injuries or health conditions, this is a program that everyone can benefit from. Every workout will have progressions and regressions so the trainee can scale up or scale down the session based on his/her ability level. Throughout the book, you will see level I, level II, and level III versions of each workout. Level I is intended for beginners who lack experience with weight-lifting technique. Level II is meant for intermediate athletes with moderate lifting experience. Level III is intended for advanced athletes with extensive experience and mastery of the major lifts. This gradient allows people to evaluate their own capacity and adjust intensity from day to day based on how their body feels.

EQUIPMENT CHECKLIST

In order to make the workouts in this book truly adaptable to a range of environments, ideally you should have access to the following pieces of equipment. Instead of opting to buy brand-name equipment, search online for DIY approaches to these workout tools. Oftentimes, you'll be able to create a durable, inexpensive version for your personal use. Above all, however, be cautious, know your limits, and test your homemade equipment thoroughly before incorporating it into your workouts.

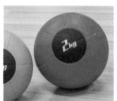

SANDBAG

Ideally, your sandbag will be refillable. This will allow you to adjust the weight of the sandbag as you progress.

Photo: Donald Chambers

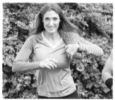

MEDICINE BALL

With a utility knife (or drill), some durable glue, and sand, you can convert an inexpensive rubber ball into your own personal medicine ball.

Photo: Shutterstock.com

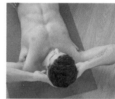

KETTLEBELL

You only need one to start. The pure iron ones are easier to grip than the rubberized ones. I suggest women begin using an 8 kg (18 lb) and men a 16 kg (35 lb).

Photo: Shutterstock.com

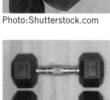

DUMBBELL

You can probably get away with three sets: a light, medium, and heavy (based on ability). Avoid adjustable dumbbells, which an add time to your workouts.

Photo: Shutterstock.com

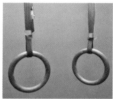

RINGS

Go with wooden rings. They're much easier to grip and last longer.

Photo: Shutterstock.com

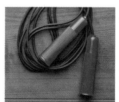

MAT

Rubber horse stall mats are the best. They're easy to clean and they never tear or wear out. Look for them at a tractor supply stores or pet stores.

Photo: Shutterstock.com

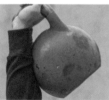

JUMP ROPE

Don't waste money on a speed rope unless you already know what you're doing. If you're just starting out, any jump rope will do.

Photo: Shutterstock.com

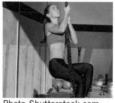

CLIMBING ROPE

Although manila ropes (the brownish ones) are cheaper, they'll make a mess and tear up your skin. Spend a little more money on a polyester fiber rope.

Photo: Shutterstock.com

USER'S GUIDE

365 WODs is a catalog of workouts divided into three categories: At Home, At the Gym, and On the Road. This way, you need never miss a workout. Keep in mind, though, that *365 WODs* is not intended to be a "cover-to-cover" training program, meaning one workout does not lead into the next. It is in no way progressive or developmental. Rather, it is a menu from which the reader must choose the appropriate workout based on his/her circumstances. This freedom will allow the creative mind to explore and experiment with hundreds of training options from day to day. It may also serve as a challenge to find a way to complete all 365 workouts.

STOPWATCH

If it starts and stops, it's good. You might try just using the clock function on your smartphone.

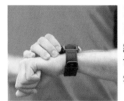

Photo:Shutterstock.com

DISCLAIMER

It is important for all readers to take time to understand the basics of the workout they intend to perform and not overstep their current ability level. A year is a long time, and progress from day to day is meant to be gradual. Do not rush to make each WOD more challenging than it needs to be.

As with any training program, *365 WODs* must be followed with caution. Movements must be meticulously learned and executed with proper technique for them to be safe and effective. All readers should begin with the regressed version of the WOD to allow the body to adapt to new movements and intensities. Plan rest days into training weeks to avoid overtraining and increasing risk of injury.

BOX

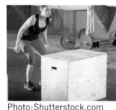

There are a lot of DIY options out there, and they aren't too difficult to build. It's definitely cheaper than buying one and having it shipped. Choose an option with

Photo:Shutterstock.com

three different heights depending on what side you rest it on—rather than one that relies on stacking. Also, wood is better on your shins than metal.

TIRE

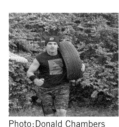

Often tractor supply stores have old tires where the tread has worn through on one side, and you'll either get it for free or really cheap. You should also

Photo:Donald Chambers

check online. But keep in mind, no two tires are the same. Before you buy it you've got to feel it to see if it's something you can flip.

GLOSSARY

1RM: one repetition maximum

6 to 1: a descending repetition scheme from the first number to the lower number

Airdyne: a version of a stationary bike that features moving handles and pedals

Air squat: a squat with no added weight

AMRAP: as many repetitions as possible

Anchor drag: move that involves dragging an object (e.g., tire, sled) behind you

Backpedal: running backwards

Ball slam: See page 45

Bear crawl (standard): See page 32

Bicycle crunches: ab crunch when you bring your opposite elbow to the opposite knee from a supine position on the floor

Box jump (standard): See page 20

Broad jump: a two-footed forward jump

Burpee (standard): See page 21

Burpee broad jump: instead of jumping vertically and clapping your hands to finish your burbee, you jump forward for distance

Butt kickers: running in place and bringing your heal up to your butt with each stride

Car push: put it in neural and—yes—push a car

Candlestick: when you gain momentum before rolling forward by rolling backwards and lifting your hips and legs towards the ceiling

Clean and jerk (advanced): See page 17

Complex: a combination of exercises done directly one after the other as a single set

Crab walk: See page 33

Dead hangs: hanging from a bar or object with straight arms

Deadlift (standard): See page 11

Deck squat: when you roll from your back into a squatting motion and stand up

Deficit deadlifts: when you elevate your feet on a block while the weight remains on the ground

Double under: a jump rope passes two times per jump

Downward facing dog: popular yoga position in which the body moves into an inverted V shape, with your buttocks in the air and your hands and feet on the ground

Duck walk: walking while in a low squat

Eccentric: lowering of a bar to the chest

EMOTM: every minute on the minute

Farmer's carry: carrying objects (often dumbbells) in your hands, one on each side, simulating pushing a wheelbarrow

Floor press: See page 37

Forward/backward roll: a somersault

Frog hop: hopping from low squat to low squat

Front squat (standard): See page 14

Full bridge: when the athlete has his or her feet and hands on the ground with his or her torso suspended upward

Glute ham raise: when an athlete follows a back extension with a leg curl

Goblet squat (standard): See page 15

Good mornings (standard): See page 31

Handstand pushup (advanced): See page 26

Hip bridge: when the athlete has his or her feet and shoulders on the ground with the torso suspended upwards

Hollow rock: See page 39

Hurdle hops: two-footed jump over a low object

Inchworm pushup: when you reach for the ground from a standing position and walk your hands forward until you reach a pushup position and then inch your feet forward toward your hands until you are able to stand again

Inchworm walk: when you walk your hands out to full-body extension and then walk your feet toward your hands while keeping your legs straight

Inverted row (standard): See page 28

Kettleball snatch: See page 38

Kettlebell swing (standard): See page 30

Kip swing: See page 47

Kipping pullup (advanced): See page 23

Kipping: a handstand pushup that uses the legs to generate upward momentum

L sit: See page 49

Lateral toes to bar: similar to a standard toes to bar except the toes contact the bar outside the grip on alternating sides

Low crawl: crawling on knees and elbows

Low dip support: the bottom position of a ring dip

Man makers: with dumbbells in each hand in a pushup position, row each dumbbell up (alternating) to your chest while doing a pushup

Man on fire burpees: when you roll between burpees

Mountain climber: See page 41

Muscle up: See page 51

Overhead squat (standard): See page 16

Parallettes: portable training tool for the parallel bars, usually made of PVC piping (see page 49)

Piked pushups: pushups done with feet or knees resting on a bench and torso as close to vertical as possible

Pistol: a squat done on one leg

Press (standard): See page 12

Push press: See page 36

Pushup (standard): See page 24

Rack pull deadlift: a deadlift that begins below the knee with the bar supported on a rack or elevated surface

Reverse burpees: when an athlete performs a deck squat and then a wall handstand

Ring dips: See page 48

Ring row: a pullup performed while holding onto the rings with your feet on the floor, leaning back at a 45-degree angle

Ring swing: See page 46

Romanian deadlift: a straight-leg version of the deadlift

Rope climb: See page 50

Sandbag squat: when you perform a squat with a sandbag on your shoulder or behind your neck

Seat roll: See page 42

Shuttle run: down-and-back running sprints

Single under: a jump rope passes one time per jump

Situp (standard): See page 25

Skin the cat: when you pass your hips through the rings in a backward tuck while holding on to the rings then return your hips to the starting position once the hips pass below head level

Sled rows: rowing the weight toward the body while facing the sled, then backing up to repeat

Sledgehammer strike: Overhead strike with a sledgehammer onto a tire or similar object, simulating a wood chopping motion

Snatch (advanced): See page 18

Split jerk: See page 35

Split squat: a one-legged squat where the leg not bearing weight is positioned a few steps behind you

Squat (standard): See page 13

Strict pullup (standard): See page 22

Suitcase carry: a walk in which you hold a weight in one hand by your side, shoulders squared, to imitate carrying a suitcase

Sumo deadlift high pull: See page 44

Superman rock: See page 40

Tabata: when you give 80 percent effort or greater for 20 seconds, then rest for 10 seconds

Thruster: See page 43

Toes to bar (standard): See page 27

Unbroken set: All reps must be completed consecutively without resting in between sets

V sit: when you begin lying on your back and fold your body in half, touching your hands to your feet at the top

Waiter's walk: a walk with one arm and weight overhead

Walking lunge (standard): See page 19

Wall ball (standard): See page 29

Wall walk: See page 34

Wheelbarrow: partner exercise where one partner holds the feet of her partner in a pushup position and walks forward, mimicking a wheelbarrow

WOD: workout of the day

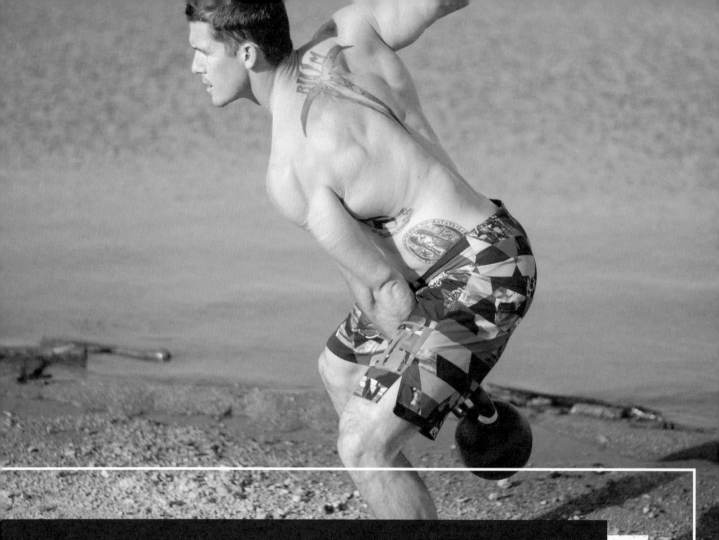

LEARN THE MOVES

These are the most common moves you'll find throughout *365 WODs.* By mastering these
basic movements, you can perform any workout in the book.

DEADLIFT (STANDARD)

1. Start with the body as close to the object as possible. If it's stone or a stump, straddle it. If it's a barbell, place the feet hip width apart with the shins lightly touching the bar.

2. Draw air into the stomach and pinch the shoulder blades together as you bend at the knees and waist to lower your hands to the object (just outside the hips for a barbell). At no time should the knees move in front of the toes or the hips be higher than the shoulders, nor should the spine be rounded.

3. Keeping the weight on the heels of the foot, push downward into the ground with your legs until the object rises to the knees. Once the object is past the knees, extend the hips and torso to a fully upright position and exhale.

4. The finish position should show the ankles, knees, hips, and shoulders in the same vertical plane. At no time should the head and neck be craned upward or downward.

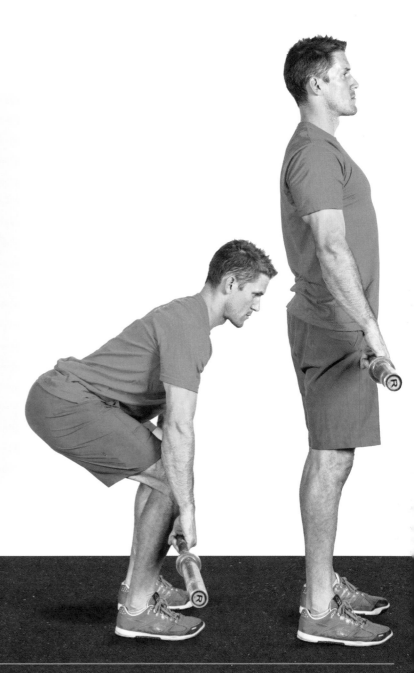

PRESS (STANDARD)

1. **Start with the object in a front rack position with the elbows beneath or slightly in front and hands at shoulder width.** Draw air into the stomach while squeezing the glutes and quadriceps, forming a solid base from which to press.

2. **Push the weight directly upward, consciously keeping it as close to the face as possible without touching.** As the weight rises above the face, force the head forward so that the arms can lock out more effectively.

3. **The finish position should show ankles, knees, hips, shoulders, elbows, and wrists all stacked in the vertical plane.**

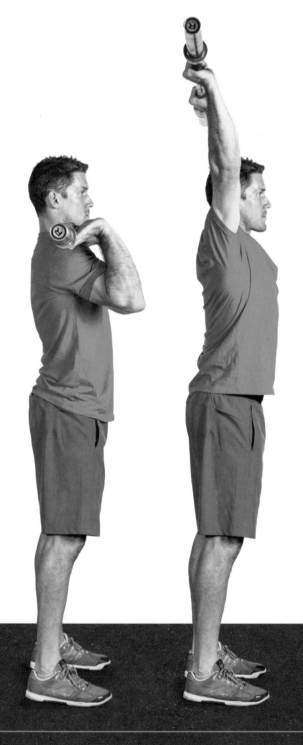

SQUAT (STANDARD)

1. Start with the feet shoulder width apart and facing forward. If you have inflexible ankles, elevate your heels by sliding a thin object underneath them. Draw air into the stomach.

2. Begin the descent by pushing the hips backward slightly, then widening the knees so that they track just on the outer edge of the feet. Your arms can be used as a counterbalance by reaching them out in front of you.

3. Keeping the torso upright, continue lowering until the top of the hip passes below the top of the knee. Push into the ground with the legs, keeping the heels in contact with the floor and stand to a fully upright position. At no time should the knees track inside of the feet.

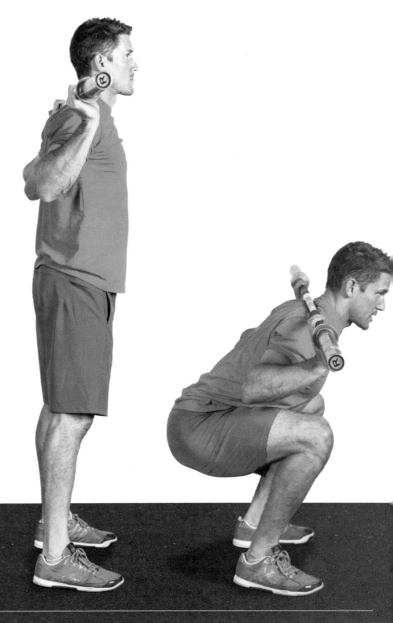

FRONT SQUAT (STANDARD)

1. **Load the bar above the collar bone with the fingers tucked just underneath for support. The higher you can raise your elbows, the better.** Start with the feet shoulder width apart and facing forward. If you have inflexible ankles, elevate your heels by sliding a thin object underneath them. Draw air into the stomach.

2. **Begin the descent by pushing the hips backward slightly, then widening the knees so that they track just on the outer edge of the feet.**

3. **Keeping the torso upright, continue lowering until the top of the hip passes below the top of the knee.** Push into the ground with the legs, keeping the heels in contact with the floor and stand to a fully upright position. At no time should the knees track inside of the feet.

The fundamentals of squatting do not change when adding weight; they adjust only for the placement of the load. If loaded in front, expect a more upright squat using the quadriceps.

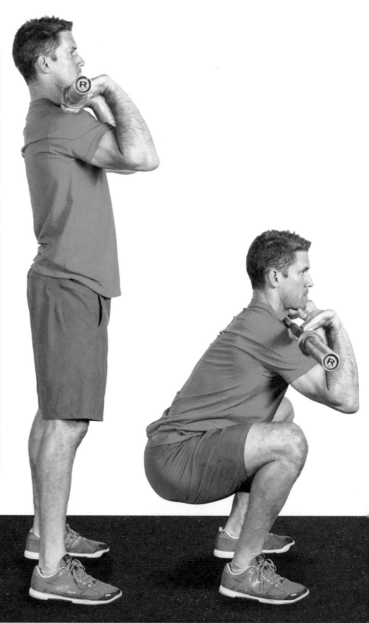

GOBLET SQUAT (STANDARD)

1. Hold the object just in front of your face with the elbows pointing down. Start with the feet shoulder width apart and facing forward. If you have inflexible ankles, elevate your heels by sliding a thin object underneath them. Draw air into the stomach.

2. Begin the descent by pushing the hips backward slightly, then widening the knees so that they track just on the outer edge of the feet.

3. Keeping the torso upright, continue lowering until the top of the hip passes below the top of the knee. Push into the ground with the legs, keeping the heels in contact with the floor and stand to a fully upright position. At no time should the knees track inside of the feet.

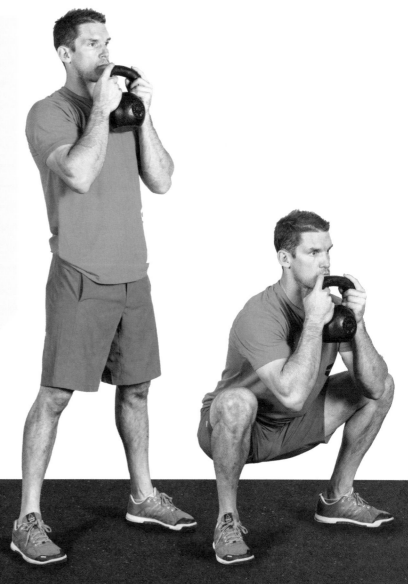

OVERHEAD SQUAT (STANDARD)

If loaded overhead, expect the upper body to pitch forward slightly during the descent. The elbows must remain locked at all times and the bar should stay just behind the vertical plane of the head throughout the movement. The wider the grip on the bar, the easier your overhead squat will be.

1. Start with the feet shoulder width apart and facing forward. If you have inflexible ankles, elevate your heels by sliding a thin object underneath them. Draw air into the stomach.

2. Begin the descent by pushing the hips backward slightly, then widening the knees so that they track just on the outer edge of the feet.

3. Continue lowering until the top of the hip passes below the top of the knee. Push into the ground with the legs, keeping the heels in contact with the floor and stand to a fully upright position. At no time should the knees track inside of the feet.

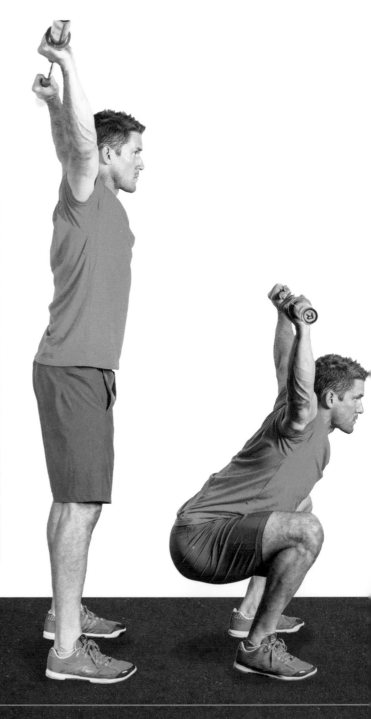

CLEAN AND JERK (ADVANCED)

1. Begin in the same fashion as the deadlift. However, as the bar passes the knees, jump and shrug the weight upward, keeping the arms relaxed and the wrists above the bar.

2. As it begins to float upward, widen the feet to a shoulder width and drop into a front squat and push the elbows aggressively forward of the bar, allowing it to settle between the shoulders and neck. The depth of the squat is determined by necessity.

3. Stand and reset your feet to hip width. Keeping the elbows high and the chest upright, draw air into the stomach and dip the knees just enough to drive the bar vertically upward.

4. Again, as the bar begins to float upward, widen the feet to shoulder width and drop just low enough to lock the elbows and wrists overhead.

5. Stand to finish from this position, bringing the feet back to hip width.

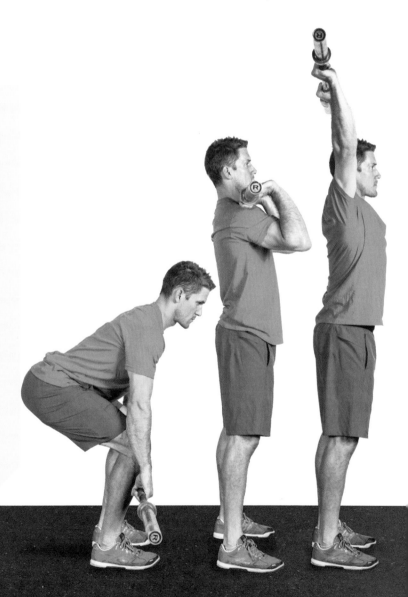

SNATCH (ADVANCED)

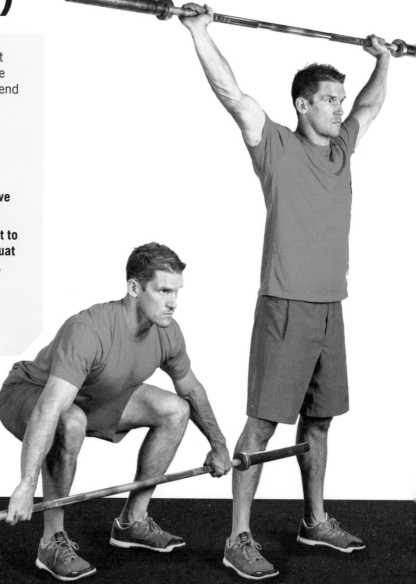

Establish a proper grip by holding the bar at waist height, then widening the hands to the point where the elbows no longer need to bend to keep the bar at the hip crease.

1. Begin in the same fashion as the deadlift (page 11).

2. As the bar passes the knees, lean back, jumping and shrugging the weight upward, keeping the arms relaxed and the wrists above the bar.

3. As it begins to float upward, widen the feet to shoulder width and drop into an overhead squat with the elbows locked aggressively upward. The depth of the squat is determined by necessity.

4. Stand and reset your feet to hip width.

WALKING LUNGE (STANDARD)

1. Put your hands on your hips. Place one foot a full stride length in front of the other and lower the back knee to the ground, allowing front and back legs to create a 90-degree angle with the ground. Your front leg will bear the majority of the weight, with that heel never leaving the ground.

2. Pull through the front heel to a standing position before placing the opposite foot in front. At no time should feet be close and directly in front of one another as if on a tightrope. Maintain normal width throughout.

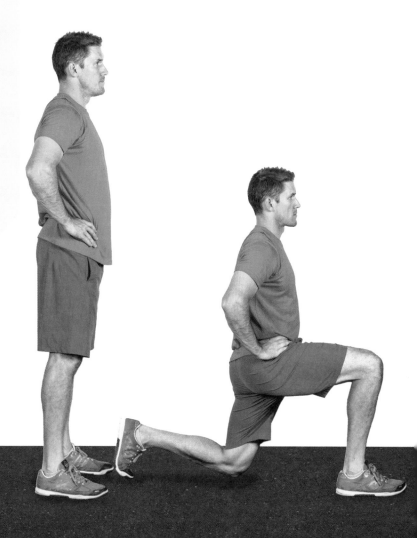

BOX JUMP (STANDARD)

1. **Stand with feet hip width apart approximately 12 inches (30.5 cm) from the object you are jumping.** The higher the object, the further away you will need to stand.

2. **Initiate the movement by swinging the arms from back to front to help generate momentum.**

3. **As the arms come forward, bend the knees slightly and jump up and onto the object.**

4. **Land with the feet hip width apart and stand to a fully upright position to finish.**

5. **Hop or step down and repeat.**

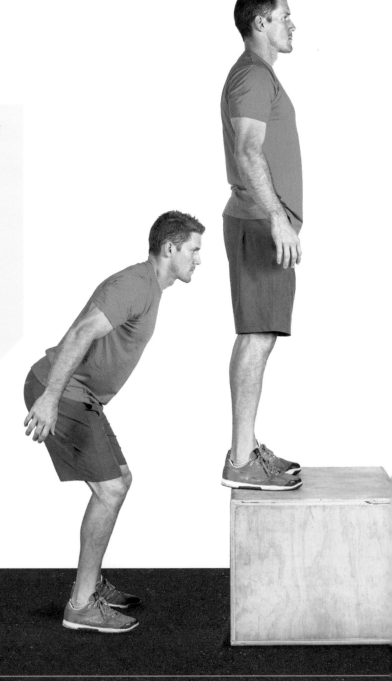

BURPEE (STANDARD)

1. **Start in a standing position. Lower the body to a prone position on the ground by either stepping or jumping the feet backward.** The entire body must be in contact with the ground at this point.

2. **By any means necessary, get the body back to a standing position.**

3. **Finish by jumping and clapping overhead at the top.**

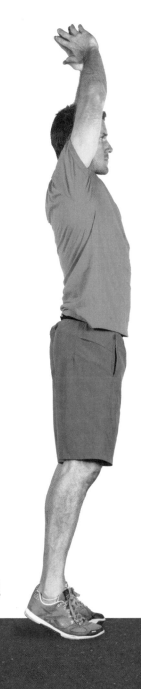

STRICT PULLUP (STANDARD)

1. Hang from the object with the hands shoulder width apart and arms straight.

2. Using the back and arms, pull the body upward until the chin is fully above the object.

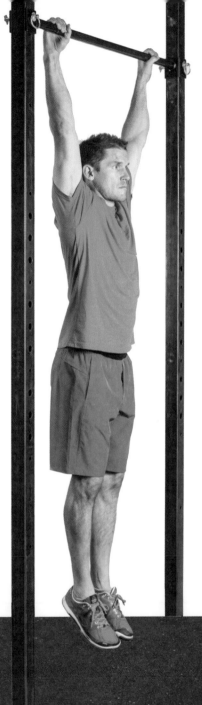

KIPPING PULLUP (ADVANCED)

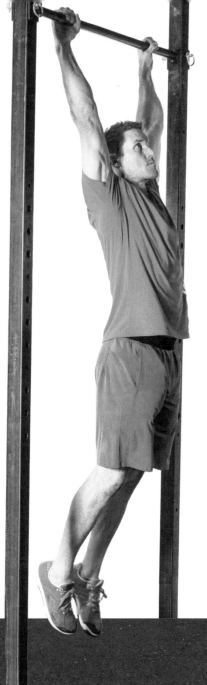

1. **Hanging from the object with the hands shoulder width apart, arms straight, and shoulder blades pinched, generate horizontal momentum by quickly moving the stomach forward and backward like a pendulum while keeping the legs straight and tight.**

2. **On the backward swing of the stomach, pump the knees quickly upward and thrust the hips forward.** This should translate the horizontal momentum into upward movement.

3. **As the body travels up, use the back and arms to pull yourself upward until the chin is clearly above the object.**

PUSHUP (STANDARD)

1. **Start with the hands shoulder width apart, feet together, and elbows straight.**

2. **Lower the chest toward the ground while keeping the elbows close to your sides and the stomach rigid and tight.** At no time should the elbows be closer to the head than the shoulders, or the hips be lower than the chest.

3. **Continue to lower the body until the chest and chin touch the ground simultaneously.**

4. **Press the hands into the ground and extend the arms using your chest and triceps until the elbows return to a fully locked position.**

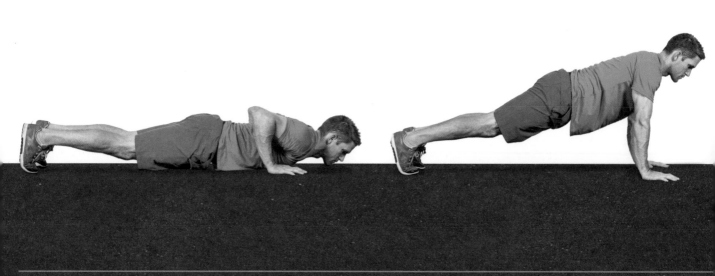

SITUP (STANDARD)

1. **Begin in a supine position on the ground with the feet together, legs straight, and arms overhead.** If you have issues with your lumbar spine, a rolled-up towel or yoga mat can be used as support in the small of the back.

2. **Keeping the feet on the ground and legs straight, pull your arms toward your waist to generate forward momentum.**

3. **Contract the stomach by pulling the belly button inward and lift the torso off the ground.**

4. **Finish by folding forward until the hands touch the feet.**

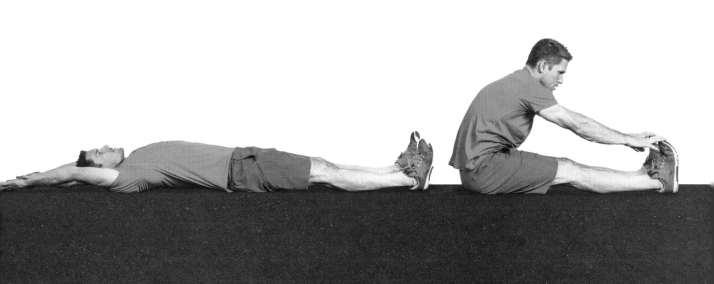

HANDSTAND PUSHUP (ADVANCED)

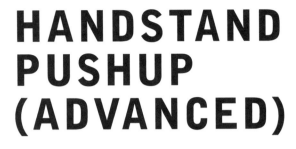

1. Begin in a handstand position against a wall or an object with arms locked and feet together. Hands should be approximately 12 inches (30.5 cm) away from the wall.

2. Lower the head toward the ground to a point 6 inches (15 cm) from the wall, continuing to reach the feet toward the sky and keeping the elbows from flaring outside the hands.

3. Without losing tension, push the ground away from you until the elbows are again locked and the body is in a full handstand.

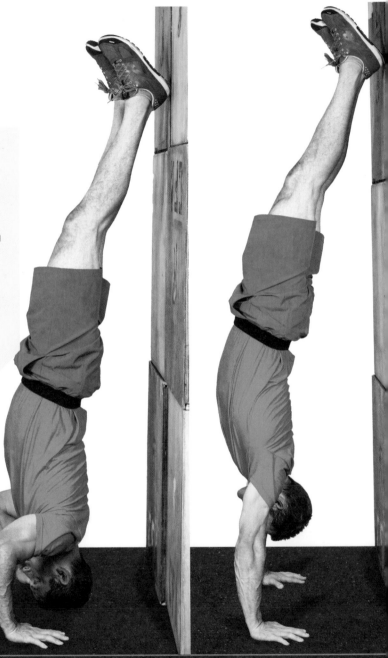

TOES TO BAR (STANDARD)

1. Hang from the object with hands shoulder width apart and arms straight.

2. Contract the stomach by pulling the belly button inward and lift the legs and hips toward the bar.

3. Keeping the arms straight throughout, lift until both feet touch the bar inside your hands.

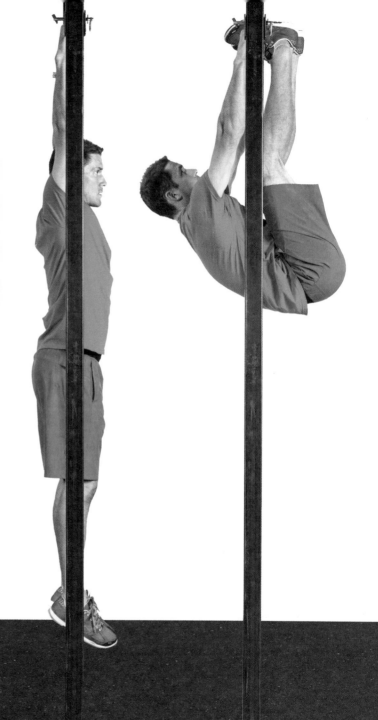

INVERTED ROW (STANDARD)

1. **With feet together on the ground, grab onto the rings or bar with both hands and lean backward away from them until the arms are straight and the body is fully suspended.** It will look like an upside-down pushup at this point.

2. **With the shoulder blades pinched, the stomach tight, and the glutes squeezed, use the back and arms to pull your chest toward the rings or bar.** At no time should the hips or knees bend.

3. **Finish by touching the chest to the bar or the rings to your ribs.**

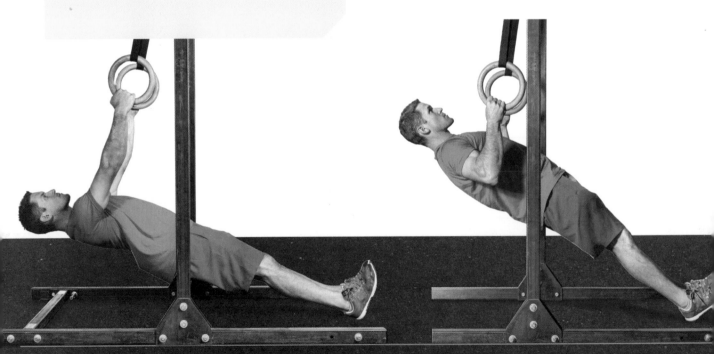

WALL BALL (STANDARD)

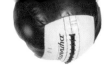

1. Start with a medicine ball in front of your face while in a standing position with feet shoulder width apart and approximately 24 inches (61 cm) away from the wall.

2. Keeping the ball in the same position, lower yourself into a full squat using proper technique.

3. As you rebound out of the squat, use the momentum gained to throw the ball up and forward until it strikes the target (10 feet [3 m] for men, 9 feet [2.7 m] for women).

4. Catch the ball in the same position as you began.

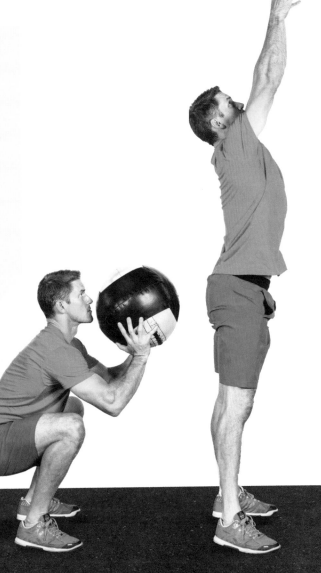

KETTLEBELL SWING (STANDARD)

1. **With the feet shoulder width apart or slightly wider, deadlift the kettlebell to a standing position.** Hands should be palms down and right next to each other on the handle.

2. **Keeping the arms straight and the weight on the heels, move the hips back and forth to create momentum.**

3. **As the hips come forward, they should push the kettlebell away from the body like a pendulum.**

4. **At the end of every swing, the kettlebell should return to the same position just under the hips, between the thighs.**

5. **As your hips generate more momentum, swing the kettlebell high enough to lock elbows and wrists with the bell directly overhead in the vertical plane.** This should remain a continuous and fluid movement, and at no time should the hips be higher than the head, or the spine be rounded.

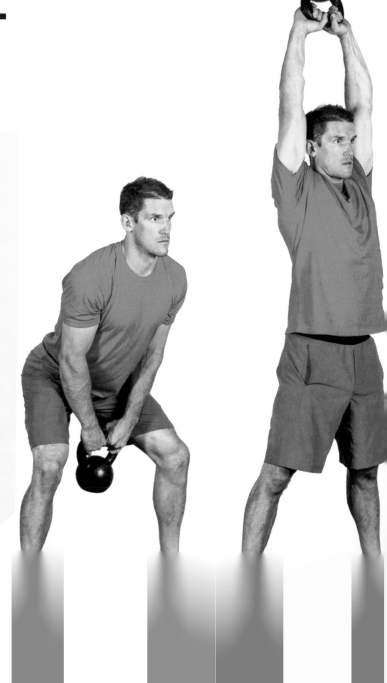

GOOD MORNINGS (STANDARD)

1. **Start with feet at hip width and hands behind the head.**

2. **Keeping your weight on your heels and knees slightly bent, shift your hips backward until the hamstrings begin to tighten.** At no time should the spine round forward.

3. **When you feel the hamstrings tighten, pull the hips forward until you return to a fully upright position.**

Adding weight to this exercise does not change the fundamental technique of it, only the placement of the load. Most commonly the weight will be loaded across the back similarly to a back squat.

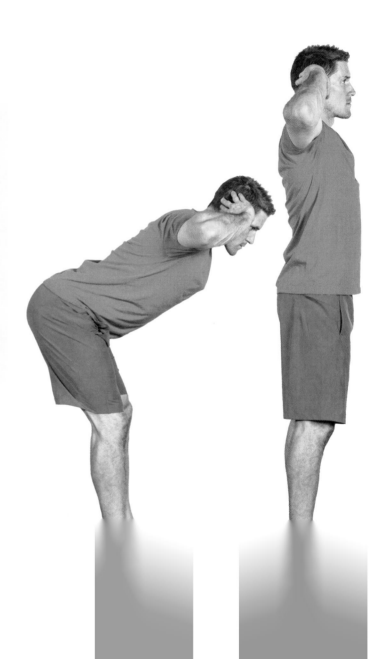

BEAR CRAWL (STANDARD)

1. Starting in a pushup position, move the right foot and left arm simultaneously forward in a crawling motion. Repeat with the left foot and right arm. The arms should remain locked out at all times while the legs can bend as needed. At no time should all the weight be on the arms or the legs.

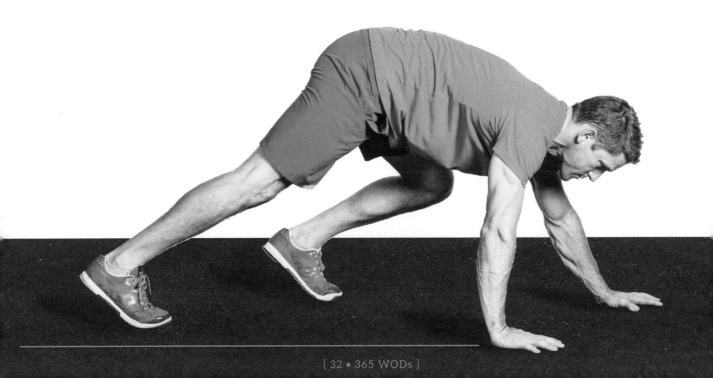

CRAB WALK

1. Starting on your butt with your hands behind you, lift your hips so that only your feet and hands are touching the ground. Move forward, backward, or sideways in this position, keeping the elbows locked the entire time.

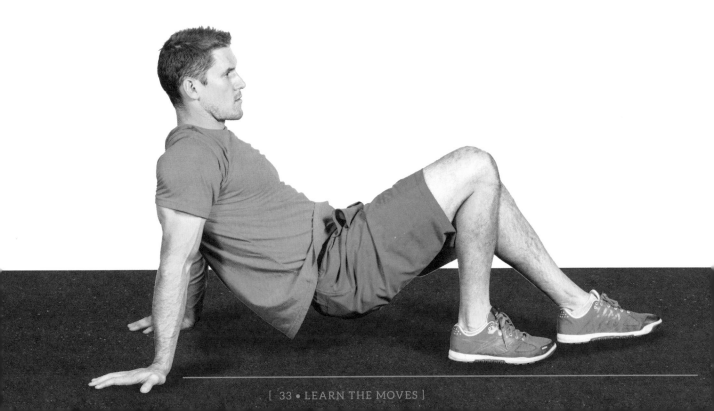

WALL WALK

1. Begin with your feet against the wall in a prone position.

2. Push your chest off the ground while reaching one foot upward toward the wall.

3. As soon as the foot plants on the wall, lift your hips over your head and place the other foot against the wall. At this point, you should be inverted to some degree.

4. Keeping the elbows locked, begin walking your hands toward the wall and your feet toward the ceiling. Your strength level will dictate how close to the wall you travel before reversing course and walking the feet back to the ground.

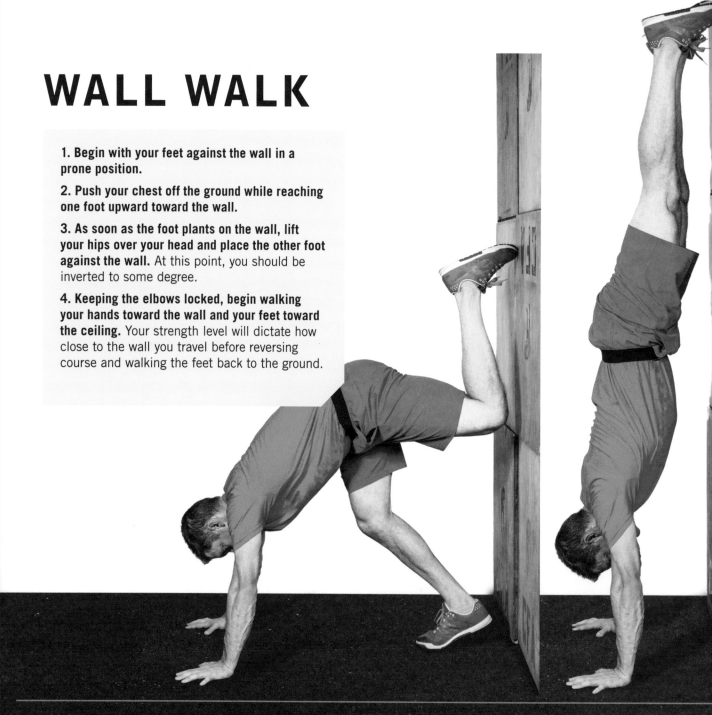

SPLIT JERK

1. Start with the bar in a front rack position.

2. Keeping your elbows at or above parallel, dip at the knees while keeping the torso upright.

3. Without pausing in the dip, jump upward while punching the bar toward the ceiling.

4. Land with one foot in front of the other, the back knee slightly bent, and the arms locked out strong overhead.

5. Bring the feet back together before bringing the bar down to the front rack.

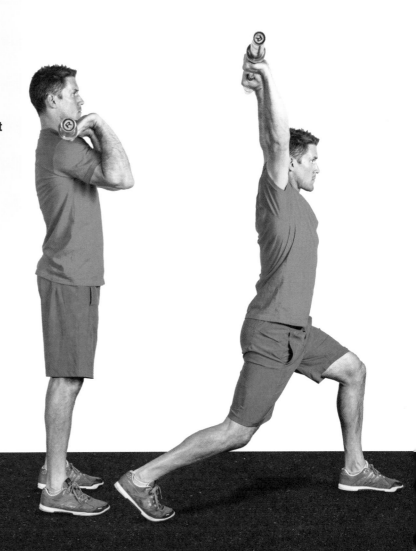

PUSH PRESS

1. Start with the bar in a front rack position.

2. Keeping your elbows at or above parallel, dip at the knees while keeping the torso upright.

3. Without pausing in the dip, drive the body and bar upward until the arms are locked overhead. Your feet should not leave the ground.

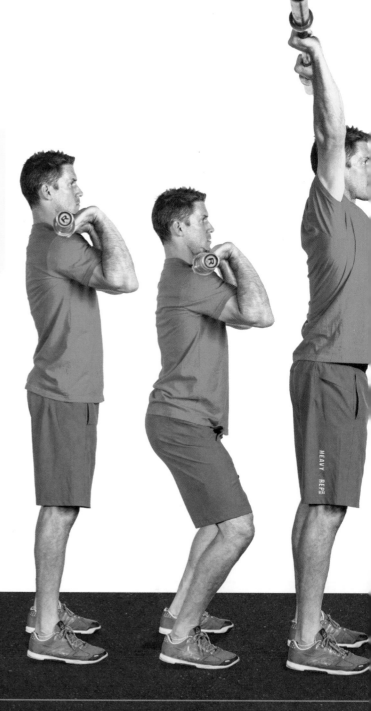

FLOOR PRESS

1. Starting supine on the floor, get your body in a position beneath the rack so your eyes are even with the bar.

2. Take the bar from the rack with arms extended and hold it in a position directly above the sternum.

3. Slowly lower the bar until both elbows touch the floor, then press firmly upward until the elbows fully lock.

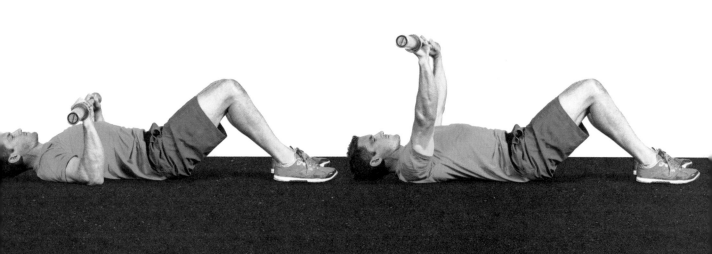

KETTLEBELL SNATCH

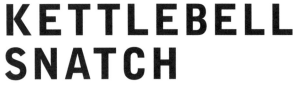

1. This is a single arm movement. Start with the kettlebell in one hand standing upright.

2. Swing the kettlebell from under the hips up and out away from the body.

3. As it starts traveling upward, pull the bell toward your face while rotating it away from the midline. At this point, it should be traveling in the diagonal plane.

4. Complete the movement by punching the hand toward the ceiling and locking the elbow and wrist into place.

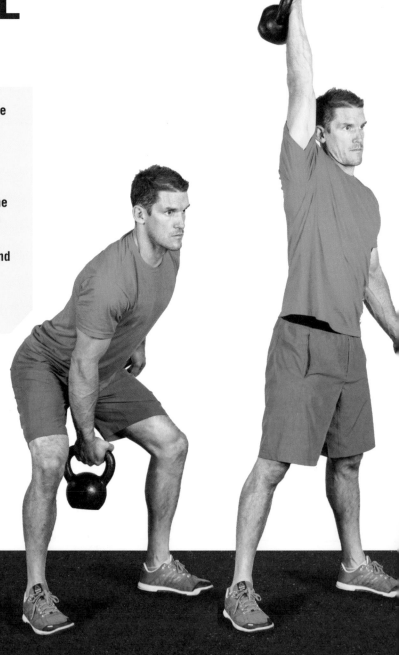

HOLLOW ROCK

1. **Starting in a supine position on the floor with arms outstretched, raise the feet and shoulders slightly off the ground.** This is your hollow body position. It may help to tuck the chin.

2. **Holding this position tightly, begin rocking the body forward and back.** Never touch the heels or the shoulder blades to the ground.

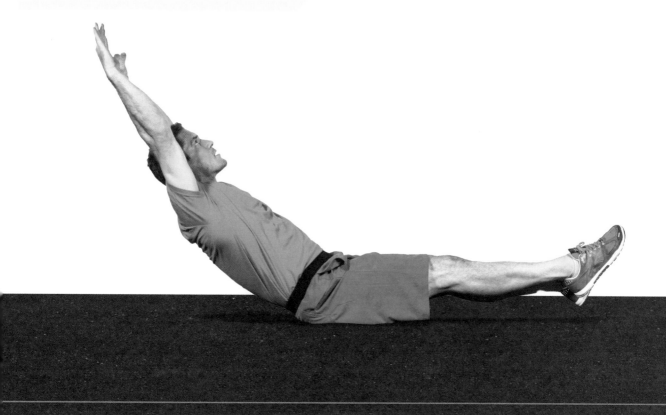

SUPERMAN ROCK

1. **Starting in a prone position on the floor with arms outstretched, raise the feet and chest slightly off the ground.** This is your Superman arch position.

2. **Holding this position tightly, begin rocking your body forward and back. Never touch the ground with your toes or your chest.**

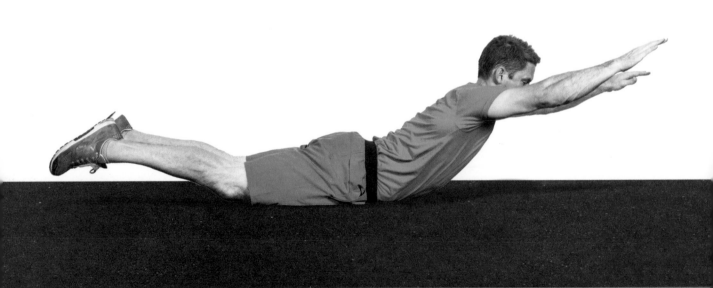

MOUNTAIN CLIMBER

1. Start in a pushup position with one knee tucked to your chest.

2. Quickly alternate which knee is tucked to the chest for the prescribed number of repetitions.

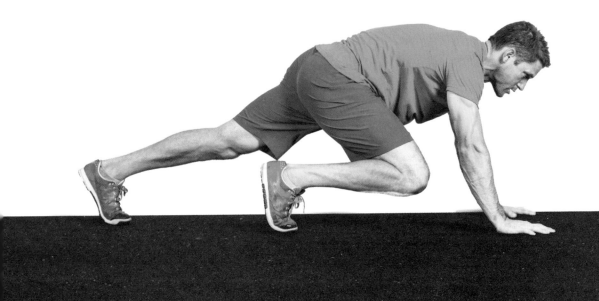

SEAT ROLL

1. Starting on your butt with your hands behind you, roll to the left or right into a pushup position.

2. Continue rolling in the same direction until you find yourself back on your butt with your hands behind.

3. Repeat in the opposite direction.

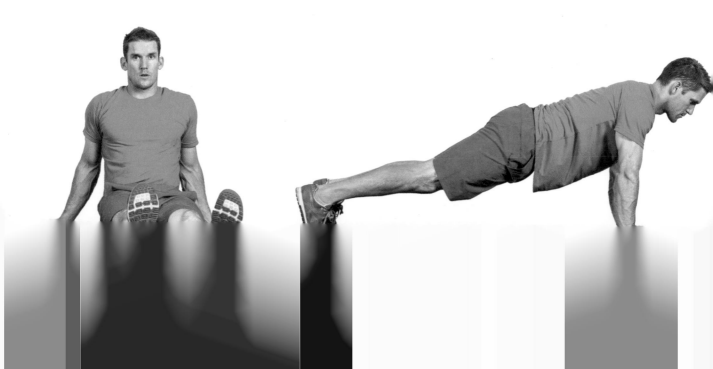

THRUSTER

1. **Begin with the bar in a front rack position with elbows at or above parallel.**

2. **Descend into a full-depth front squat.**

3. **As you come to the top of the squat, begin pressing the bar overhead until it is fully locked.** This should feel like the seamless combination of a front squat and a push press.

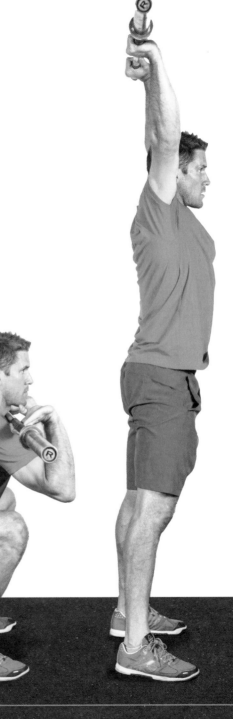

SUMO DEADLIFT HIGH PULL

1. With the feet set wide apart, take the bar with a narrow grip.

2. Deadlift it off the ground in this position and raise it to your collarbone without pausing. The elbows should stay above the wrists at all times.

3. Return the bar to the hanging position immediately and then lower the bar to the ground.

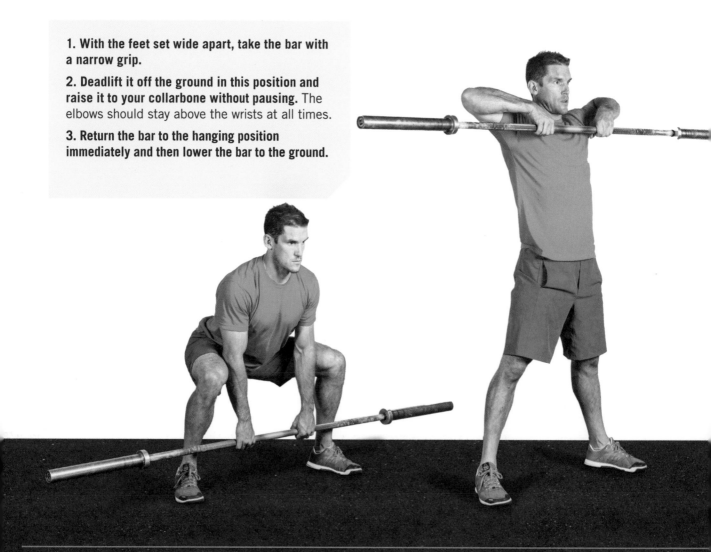

BALL SLAM

1. Begin with the ball on the ground between your feet. Squat down to pick it up in both hands and raise it overhead in one fluid motion.

2. As soon as you hit full extension of the arms above the head, slam the ball back to the ground between your feet.

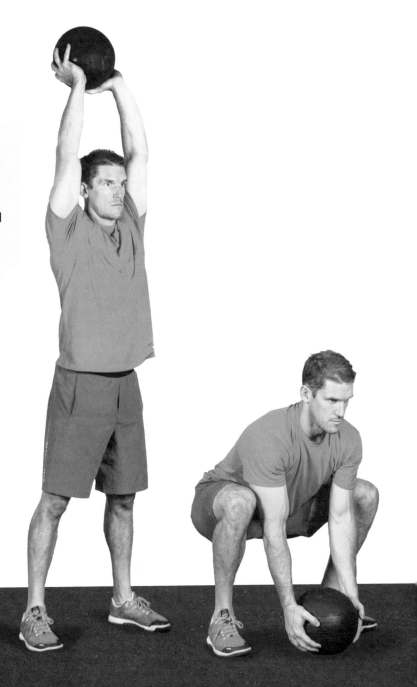

RING SWING

1. Begin by hanging from the rings with arms and legs extended.

2. Slowly move your body back and forth between a hollow position and an arched position.

3. As you hit the hollow position, pull the rings slightly backward. As you hit the arched position, push the rings slightly forward.

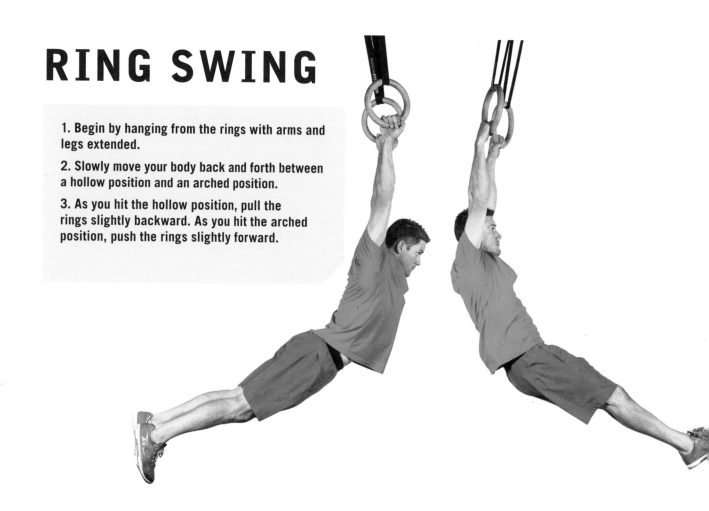

KIP SWING

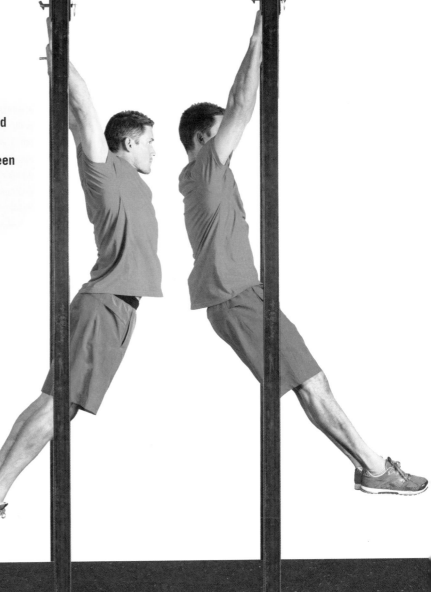

1. Begin by hanging from the bar with arms and legs extended.

2. Slowly move your body back and forth between a hollow position and an arched position.

RING DIPS

1. Begin with the elbows locked out above the rings and the arms tucked tightly to your sides.

2. Keeping the rings close to the sides, tilt the chest and shoulders forward and down until the arms touch the top of the rings.

3. Reverse the movement by pressing firmly downward until you return to a fully locked position above the rings.

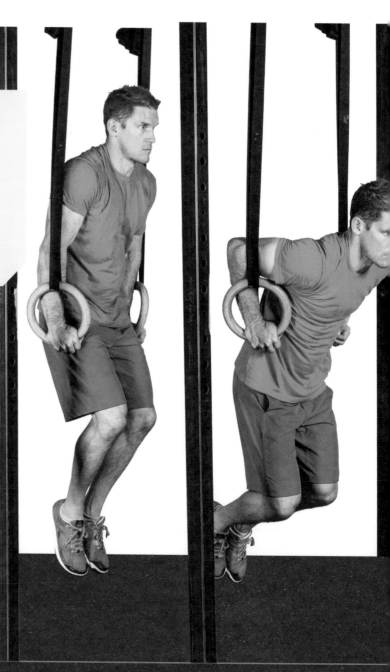

L SIT

1. Keeping the legs as straight as possible, lift them off the ground while keeping the rest of your body totally neutral. This can be done hanging from a bar or by supporting your weight on parallel bars or something similar.

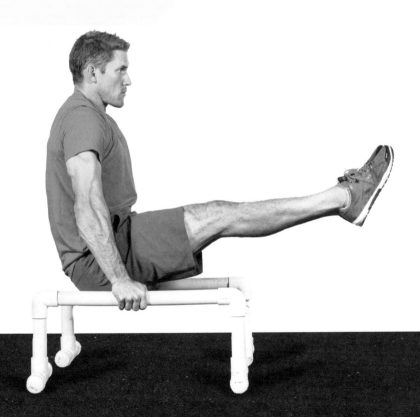

ROPE CLIMB

There are many variations on how to climb a rope. (1) Legless refers to a climb without the use of the legs or feet. (2) A standard rope climb refers to a climb utilizing a foot or leg lock technique to assist the ascent. (3) A climb to standing begins with in the supine position with the rope hanging above.

1. Keeping the legs as straight as possible, pull upright to a standing position.

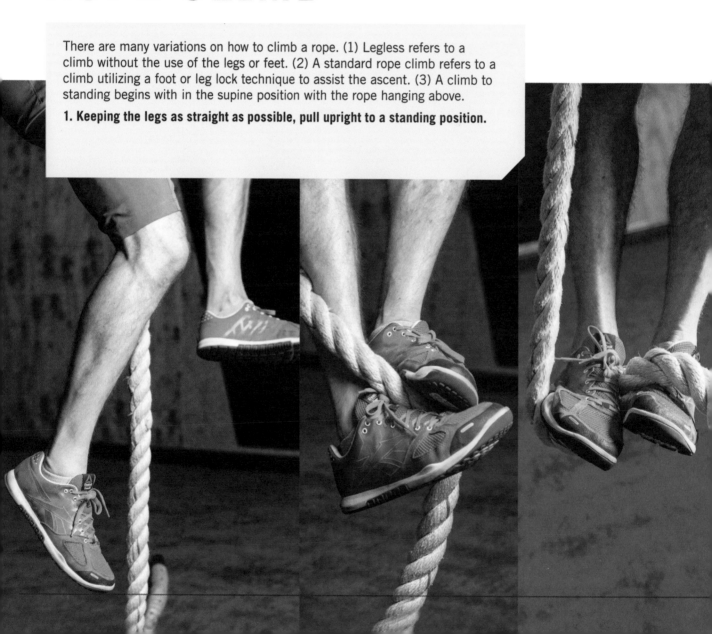

MUSCLE UP

1. **Start by hanging on the rings/bar with arms and legs extended.**

2. **Kip or ring swing to gain momentum, then forcefully thrust your hips upward toward the rings/bar.** The hips should be the highest point of the body and the arms should remain as straight as possible.

3. **At this exact moment, throw your head forward and through the rings (over the bar), catching yourself in a dip position.**

4. **Once stabilized, press out the dip until both arms are locked and you are in a supported position above the rings/bar.**

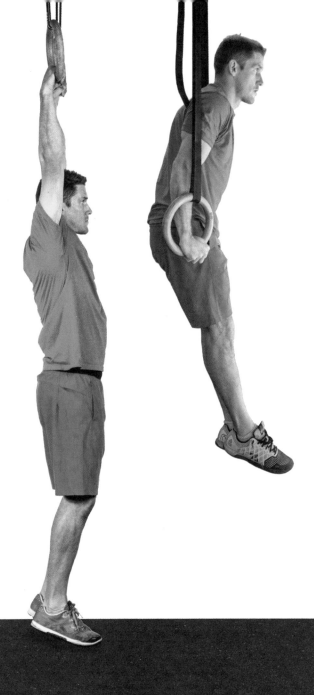

CHAPTER 1
WODs at Home

This section is dedicated to workouts that can be performed in your home or in your neighborhood. Because every home is different, I've included elements that allow you to take advantage of any style of home or neighborhood, with workouts using walls, streets, steps, etc. But if a workout requires a swimming pool and you don't have one, skip it and move on to the next one. Certain workouts will also require some basic portable equipment like gymnastics rings, a jump rope, or a refillable sandbag. If you do not have access to these, substitute something similar.

001

LEVEL I
5-x-400-meter sprints
Rest 5 minutes between efforts

LEVEL II
5-x-400-meter sprints
Rest 5 minutes between efforts

LEVEL III
5-x-400-meter sprints
Rest 5 minutes between efforts

NOTES: "Sprint" should be understood as 90 percent effort unless you have been sprinting regularly.

002

LEVEL I
¼-mile (400 m) swim +
1-mile (1.6 km) run

LEVEL II
For time:
½-mile (800 m) swim + 2-mile
(3.2 km) run

LEVEL III
For time:
1-mile (1.6 km) swim + 2-mile
(3.2 km) run

NOTES: This is an aerobic effort, so pace it slowly. Swim can be done in a pool or open water. Approximate distances are okay.

"For time" means you should track the time it takes to complete the WOD. **"Rounds for time"** means you'll track the time it takes to complete all the rounds. This will help you gauge your progress if you repeat the WOD later on.

003

LEVEL I
20 wall walks for time
50 single unders every broken set

LEVEL II
Handstand walk 50-meters for time
20 double unders every broken set

LEVEL III
Handstand walk 100-meters for time
30 double unders every broken set

NOTES: "Single under" refers to a jump rope passing one time per jump. "Double under" refers to a jump rope passing two times per jump. Wall walks are done to each athlete's ability level. The goal is to get the chest to the wall eventually. If handstand walk is done outdoors, wear gloves.

004

LEVEL I
75 wall balls for time

LEVEL II
100 wall balls for time

LEVEL III
150 wall balls for time

NOTES: Medicine ball can be any weight. Target should be 10 feet (3 m) for men and 9 feet (2.7 m) for women.

WODs AT HOME

005

LEVEL I
5-x-50-meter swim sprints
Rest 2 minutes between efforts

LEVEL II
3-x-100-meter swim sprints
Rest 2 minutes between efforts

LEVEL III
5-x-100-meter swim sprints
Rest 2 minutes between efforts

NOTES: Pool or open water is okay. Keep strictly to
the rest periods.

006

LEVEL I
For time:
30 sandbag throws
1-mile (1.6 km) run

LEVEL II
2 rounds for time:
30 sandbag throws
1-mile (1.6 km) run

LEVEL III
3 rounds for time:
30 sandbag throws
1-mile (1.6 km) run

NOTES: Sandbags should be thrown forward from between
the legs. The distance of the throw is not important.
Sandbags can be filled to any weight.

007

LEVEL I
5 rounds for completion:
5 wall walks
:20 V sit hold

LEVEL II
5 rounds for completion:
10 wall handstand shoulder
touches
:10 L sit hold

LEVEL III
5 rounds for completion:
10 free handstand shoulder
touches
:20 L sit hold

NOTES: This is a skill test. There
is no time component, so do not
rush. L sit holds must be done from
parallettes or the ground.

"For completion"
means to focus
on form and
technique rather
than time to
complete the
WOD.

:20 = 20 seconds

008

LEVEL I
With a partner, complete the following for time in any order:
100 situps
100 pushups
100 squats

LEVEL II
With a partner, complete the following for time in any order:
150 situps
150 pushups
150 squats

LEVEL III
With a partner, complete the following for time in any order:
200 situps
200 pushups
200 squats

NOTES: Partners are not allowed to work simultaneously.
If no partner is available, cut reps in half and complete in
any order.

WODs AT HOME

009

LEVEL I
EMOTM; 10-minutes:
2 wall walks

LEVEL II
EMOTM; 10-minutes:
5-meter handstand walk

LEVEL III
EMOTM; 10-minutes:
10-meter handstand walk

NOTES: This is a skill test. There is no penalty for failing a round.

EMOTM = Every minute on the minute.

010

LEVEL I
Complete in any order:
Accumulate 3 minutes in a wall walk
Accumulate 3 minutes in a V sit
Accumulate 3 minutes in a hip bridge

LEVEL II
Complete in any order:
Accumulate 4 minutes in a wall handstand
Accumulate 4 minutes in an L sit
Accumulate 4 minutes in a bridge

LEVEL III
Complete in any order:
Accumulate 5 minutes in a free handstand
Accumulate 5 minutes in an L sit
Accumulate 5 minutes in a bridge

NOTES: This is a skill test with no speed component. Free handstands are allowed to move but not walk. Whether to bridge or hip bridge should be decided based on shoulder and thoracic flexibility. A full bridge is when the feet and hands are on the ground with the torso suspended upward. A hip bridge is when the the feet and shoulders are on the ground with the torso suspended upwards. "V sit" refers to the exercise in which you begin lying on your back and folds your body in half, touching the hands to the feet at the top.

011

LEVEL I

5 rounds for completion:
10 hollow rocks
10 air squats
10-meter bear crawl

LEVEL II

5 rounds for completion:
5 candlestick to deck squat
5 wall handstand shoulder touches each arm

LEVEL III

5 rounds for completion:
5 candlestick to pistol each leg
5 free handstand shoulder touches each arm

NOTES: This is a skill test with no time component. At level II, you may use hands to assist the deck squat. "Air squat" refers to a squat with no added weight. "Pistol" refers to a squat done on one leg. "Deck squat" is when you roll from youtr back into a squatting motion and stand up. "Candlestick" is a specific way of gaining momentum before rolling forward. It is done by rolling backward and lifting the hips and legs toward the ceiling.

012

LEVEL I

10-minute AMRAP:
200-meter run
10 ring rows
5 pushups

LEVEL II

15-minute AMRAP:
400-meter run
4 muscle ups

LEVEL III

20-minute AMRAP:
400-meter run
7 muscle ups

AMRAP = As many repetitions as possible.

NOTES: This is a high-volume workout, so pick a steady pace on the runs. At level III, you should do as many rounds of unbroken muscle ups as possible. "Ring row" is a pullup with the feet on the ground. The rings allow the athlete to adjust the angle of pull by walking their feet forward or back.

013

LEVEL I

Perform an increasing number of object swings EMOTM until failure to complete:

1 kettlebell swing

2 kettlebell swings

3 kettlebell swings

(and so forth)

LEVEL II

Perform an increasing number of object swings EMOTM until failure to complete:

1 kettlebell swing

2 kettlebell swings

3 kettlebell swings

(and so forth)

LEVEL III

Perform an increasing number of object swings EMOTM until failure to complete:

1 kettlebell swing

2 kettlebell swings

3 kettlebell swings

(and so forth)

NOTES: This workout will end upon failing to complete the number of swings required. It's important to get the work done quickly to guarantee a reasonable rest period each minute. Object can be kettlebell, dumbbell, paint can, etc. Object can be any weight. At level I do Russian-style swings (eye level). At level II and level III, do American-style swings (overhead).

014

LEVEL I

Perform an increasing number of burpees EMOTM until failure to complete:

1 burpee in minute 1

2 burpees in minute 2

3 burpees in minute 3

(and so forth)

LEVEL II

Perform an increasing number of burpees EMOTM until failure to complete:

1 burpee in minute 1

2 burpees in minute 2

3 burpees in minute 3

(and so forth)

LEVEL III

Perform an increasing number of burpees EMOTM until failure to complete:

1 burpee in minute 1

2 burpees in minute 2

3 burpees in minute 3

(and so forth)

NOTES: This workout will end upon failing to complete the number of burpees required. It's important to get the work done quickly to guarantee a reasonable rest period each minute.

015

LEVEL I
EMOTM; 10-minutes:
1 wall walk
20 single unders

LEVEL II
EMOTM; 10-minutes:
2 wall walks
20 double unders

LEVEL III
EMOTM; 10-minutes:
3 wall walks
20 double unders

NOTES: Wall walks should be done to mirror your level. At level III, touch your chest to the wall before walking back out.

016

LEVEL I
30-minute swim for distance

LEVEL II
30-minute swim for distance

LEVEL III
30-minute swim for distance

NOTES: Swim can be done in pool or open water. This is an aerobic capacity workout, so the goal is to swim continuously for 30 minutes.

WODs AT HOME

017

LEVEL I

6 rounds for completion:
100-meter sprint
5 situps
5 pushups
5 squats
Rest 2-minute between efforts

LEVEL II

8 rounds for completion:
100-meter sprint
7 situps
7 pushups
7 squats
Rest 1.5 minutes between efforts

LEVEL III

10 rounds for completion:
100-meter sprint
10 situps
10 pushups
10 squats
Rest 1-minute between efforts

NOTES: Each round is meant to be full effort. Sprints should be 90 percent effort unless you have been sprinting regularly.

018

LEVEL I

For time:
50-meter walking lunge
50-meter burpee broad jump
50-meter bear crawl
50-meter crab walk

LEVEL II

For time:
75-meter walking lunge
75-meter burpee broad jump
75-meter bear crawl
75-meter crab walk

LEVEL III

For time:
100-meter walking lunge
100-meter burpee broad jump
100-meter bear crawl
100-meter crab walk

NOTES: This is slow grind workout. None of these movements covers distance quickly, so a steady pace is recommended. If done outside, wear gloves. "Burpee broad jump" is a burpee, but instead of jumping vertically and clapping the hands, you jump forward for distance.

019

LEVEL I
3 rounds for time:
400-meter forward run
400-meter backward run

LEVEL II
4 rounds for time:
400-meter forward run
400-meter backward run

LEVEL III
5 rounds for time:
400-meter forward run
400-meter backward run

NOTES: Go to a school or park for safety on the backward run. Best option is a track.

020

LEVEL I
Accumulate 3 minutes in a headstand
Accumulate 3 minutes in low dip support
Accumulate 3 minutes in squat
Accumulate 3 minutes in downward facing dog

LEVEL II
Accumulate 4 minutes in a headstand
Accumulate 4 minutes in low dip support
Accumulate 4 minutes in squat
Accumulate 4 minutes in downward facing dog

LEVEL III
Accumulate 5 minutes in a headstand
Accumulate 5 minutes in low dip support
Accumulate 5 minutes in squat
Accumulate 5 minutes in downward facing dog

NOTES: Time may be accumulated in any order for all exercises. Goal is to finish in 40 minutes. "Low dip support" is the bottom position of a ring dip. "Downward facing dog" refers to the popular yoga position.

021

LEVEL I
200-meter car push for time

LEVEL II
400-meter car push for time

LEVEL III
800-meter car push for time

NOTES: If possible, pick a course or loop that is flat. Any sort of elevation will affect the car push.

022

LEVEL I
10-minute AMRAP:
2 wall walks
4 walking lunges
6 burpees

LEVEL II
15-minute AMRAP:
2 wall walks
4 walking lunges
6 burpees

LEVEL III
20-minute AMRAP:
2 wall walks
4 walking lunges
6 burpees

NOTES: These sets must be done quickly in order to finish them in a minute. If you fail to complete required work, you rest the following minute, then resume.

023

LEVEL I
7-minute AMRAP:
200-meter run
10 burpees

LEVEL II
7-minute AMRAP:
200-meter run
10 burpees

LEVEL III
7-minute AMRAP:
200-meter run
10 burpees

NOTES: This is not a sprint, but the pace must be fast. Attempt to operate around 80 percent effort the entire time.

024

LEVEL I
Wall walk:
Complete 1 rep EMOTM; 10 minutes

LEVEL II
Kipping handstand pushup from elevation:
Complete 1 rep EMOTM; 10 minutes

LEVEL III
Kipping handstand pushup from elevation:
Complete 5 reps EMOTM; 10 minutes

NOTES: This is a skill test. Elevation for the handstand pushups can be created with boxes, parallettes, or stones. The height of elevation depends on ability level. "Kipping" a handstand pushup refers to using the legs to generate upward momentum.

WODs AT HOME

025

LEVEL I
10-minute AMRAP:
25-meter bear crawl
25-meter squat jump

LEVEL II
12-minute AMRAP:
25-meter bear crawl
25-meter squat jump

LEVEL III
15-minute AMRAP:
25-meter bear crawl
25-meter squat jump

NOTES: The squat jumps will be very tiring, so prepare for that. Pace the bear crawls steadily to reserve energy for the jumps.

026

LEVEL I
For time:
25 squats
20 walking lunges
15 pushups
10 situps
5 wall walks
10 situps
15 pushups
20 walking lunges
25 squats

LEVEL II
For time:
40 squats
30 walking lunges
20 pushups
10 situps
5 wall walks
10 situps
20 pushups
30 walking lunges
40 squats

LEVEL III
For time:
50 squats
40 walking lunges
30 pushups
20 situps
10 wall walks
20 situps
30 pushups
40 walking lunges
50 squats

027

LEVEL I

EMOTM; 20-minutes:
10 hollow rocks
5 burpees

LEVEL II

EMOTM; 20-minutes:
10 hollow rocks
7 burpees

LEVEL III

EMOTM; 20-minutes:
10 hollow rocks
10 burpees

NOTES: This is a skill test. Move quickly on the burpees in order to complete the rounds each minute. If a minute is failed, rest the following minute and then resume.

028

LEVEL I

Perform an additional walking lunge EMOTM; until failure to complete
1 walking lunge in minute 1
2 walking lunges in minute 2
3 walking lunges in minute 3
(and so forth)

LEVEL II

Perform an additional jump lunge EMOTM; until failure to complete
1 jump lunge in minute 1
2 jump lunges in minute 2
3 jump lunges in minute 3
(and so forth)

LEVEL III

Perform 2 additional jump lunges EMOTM; until failure to complete
2 jump lunges in minute 1
4 jump lunges in minute 2
6 jump lunges in minute 3
(and so forth)

NOTES: This workout will end upon failing to complete the number of walking or jump lunges required. It's important to get the work done quickly to guarantee a reasonable rest period each minute.

029

LEVEL I
200-meter bear crawl for time
Every 50-meters perform 20 situps + 20 pushups

LEVEL II
300-meter bear crawl for time
Every 50-meters perform 20 situps + 20 pushups

LEVEL III
400-meter bear crawl for time
Every 50-meters perform 20 situps + 20 pushups

NOTES: The 50-meter increments can be approximated. The situps and pushups are meant to break up the monotony of the bear crawl but should not be treated like a rest period.

030

LEVEL I
3 rounds for time:
10 object squats
50 single unders

LEVEL II
4 rounds for time:
10 object squats
30 double unders

LEVEL III
5 rounds for time:
10 object squats
50 double unders

NOTES: Object should weigh 50 pounds (22.5 kg) or more for men and 30 pounds (13.5 kg) or more for women. It can be anything.

031

LEVEL I
For completion:
200-meter swim
3-mile (4.8 km) bike
1-mile (1.6 km) run

LEVEL II
For completion:
400-meter swim
4-mile (6.4 km) bike
1-mile (1.6 km) run

LEVEL III
For completion:
500-meter swim
5-mile (8 km) bike
2-mile (3.2 km) run

NOTES: Swims can be done in a pool or open water. If open water, distances can be approximated. Workout must be performed in the order written.

032

LEVEL I
3 rounds for completion:
3 wall walks
Forward roll to seated
Backward roll to seated

LEVEL II
4 rounds for completion:
5-meter handstand walk
Forward roll to stand
Backward roll to stand

LEVEL III
5 rounds for completion:
5-meter handstand walk
Forward roll to stand
Backward roll to handstand

NOTES: This is a skill test with no time component. Movements should be practiced for quality, not speed. "Forward/backward roll" refers to somersaults.

WODs AT HOME

033

LEVEL I
For time:
50 burpees

LEVEL II
For time:
75 burpees

LEVEL III
For time:
100 burpees

NOTE: This is a sprint.

034

LEVEL I
5 rounds for time:
100-meter run
10 pushups
10 air squats

LEVEL II
7 rounds for time:
100-meter run
15 pushups
15 air squats

LEVEL III
10 rounds for time:
100-meter run
20 pushups
20 air squats

NOTES: This is a high-volume, fast-paced workout. At level II and level III, you should be moving the entire time.

035

LEVEL I
½-mile (800 m) sandbag carry (shoulder technique)

LEVEL II
1-mile (1.6 km) sandbag carry (shoulder technique)

LEVEL III
1-mile (1.6 km) sandbag carry (bearhug technique)

NOTES: This is not for time, so don't feel the need to run unless you really want to. Shoulder technique means carrying the sandbag on the shoulders. Bearhug technique means clutching the sandbag to the chest.

036

LEVEL I
3 rounds for time:
20-meter broad jump
20-meter backpedal
20-meter inchworm pushup

LEVEL II
4 rounds for time:
20-meter broad jump
20-meter backpedal
10-meter handstand walk

LEVEL III
5 rounds for time:
20-meter broad jump
20-meter backpedal
20-meter handstand walk

NOTES: If possible, find a park or school and bring gloves. "Broad jump" refers to a two-footed forward jump. Backpedal is running backwards. Inchworm pushup is when you reach for the ground from a standing position and walk the hands forward until attaining a pushup position. After the pushup, inch the feet forward toward the hands until able to stand again.

037

LEVEL I

Perform an increasing number of object push presses EMOTM up to 15 minutes.

1 press in minute 1
2 presses in minute 2
3 presses in minute 3
(and so forth)

LEVEL II

Perform an increasing number of object push presses EMOTM up to 20 minutes.

1 press in minute 1
2 presses in minute 2
3 presses in minute 3
(and so forth)

LEVEL III

Perform an increasing number of object push presses EMOTM until failure to complete.

1 press in minute 1
2 presses in minute 2
3 presses in minute 3
(and so forth)

NOTE: Object can be a kettlebell, dumbbell, stone, branch, etc.

038

LEVEL I

10-minute AMRAP:
50-meter object drag
50-meter hand-over-hand object drag
10 burpees

LEVEL II

15-minute AMRAP:
50-meter object drag
50-meter hand-over-hand object drag
10 burpees

LEVEL III

20-minute AMRAP:
50-meter object drag
50-meter hand-over-hand object drag
10 burpees

NOTES: You will need rope for this workout. Object can be a tire, sled, etc. It must be pulled like a sled for the first 50-meters, then rowed toward the body like an anchor the next 50-meters.

039

LEVEL I
30 wall muscle ups for time

LEVEL II
40 wall muscle ups for time

LEVEL III
50 wall muscle ups for time

NOTES: Wall should be chest high or higher and may be ascended any way possible.

040

LEVEL I
2 rounds for time:
20 burpees + lateral hop
40 walking lunges
60 single unders

LEVEL II
2 rounds for time:
30 burpees + lateral hop
60 walking lunges
90 single unders

LEVEL III
3 rounds for time:
30 burpees + lateral hop
60 walking lunges
90 single unders

NOTE: Lateral hops on burpees should alternate direction every rep.

WODs AT HOME

041

LEVEL I
10-minute AMRAP:
1 wall walk
2 deck squats
3 burpees
4 squat jumps
5 good mornings

LEVEL II
12-minute AMRAP:
1 wall walk
2 deck squats
3 burpees
4 squat jumps
5 good mornings

LEVEL III
15-minute AMRAP:
1 wall walk
2 deck squats
3 burpees
4 squat jumps
5 good mornings

NOTES: The pace for this workout should be moderate. At level I and level II, use hands to assist the deck squat. Squat jumps do not need to be maximum height. Wall walks should be done to your ability level.

042

LEVEL I
3 rounds of each:
:30 plank hold
:30 squat hold
:30 wall handstand hold
:30 dead hang hold
:30 V sit hold

LEVEL II
4 rounds of each:
:45 plank hold
:45 squat hold
:45 wall handstand hold
:45 dead hang hold
:45 L sit hold

LEVEL III
5 rounds of each:
1-minute plank hold
1-minute squat hold
1-minute wall handstand hold
1-minute dead hang hold
1-minute L sit hold

NOTES: It is okay to break up the planks, squats, handstands, dead hangs, and L sits into multiple sets if you cannot hold them the entire time. But squats cannot not start until planks are finished, handstands cannot start until squats are finished, etc. Dead hangs refer to hanging from a bar or object with straight arms

043

LEVEL I
For time:
50 pushups
50 bicycle crunches
50 seat rolls
50 walking lunges

LEVEL II
For time:
75 pushups
75 bicycle crunches
75 seat rolls
75 walking lunges

LEVEL III
For time:
100 pushups
100 bicycle crunches
100 seat rolls
100 walking lunges

NOTES: This is a high-volume endurance workout.
Exercises must be completed in the order listed. Bicycle
crunches are when the opposite elbow is brought to the
opposite knee from a supine position.

044

LEVEL I
3 rounds for time:
10 object squats
10 object push presses

LEVEL II
4 rounds for time:
12 object squats
12 object push presses

LEVEL III
5 rounds for time:
15 object squats
15 object push presses

NOTES: Object can be any household item weighing 20
pounds (9 kg) or more. Squats can be done in any fashion.

WODs AT HOME

045

LEVEL I
3 rounds for time:
400-meter run
:30 plank hold
:30 hip bridge hold

LEVEL II
4 rounds for time:
400-meter run
:45 plank hold
:45 hip bridge hold

LEVEL III
5 rounds for time:
400-meter run
1:00 plank hold
1:00 hip bridge hold

046

LEVEL I
100-meter backward car push for time

LEVEL II
200-meter backward car push for time

LEVEL III
300-meter backward car push for time

NOTES: The 100-meter course should be flat and the athlete should be walking backward with his/her back against the car

047

LEVEL I
21-15-9-for time:
Object deadlift
Hand release pushups
Hollow rocks

LEVEL II
21-15-9-for time:
Object deadlift
Piked pushups
Situps

LEVEL III
21-15-9-for time:
Object deadlift
Handstand pushups
Situps

NOTES: Object can be anything weighing more than 100 pounds (45.5 kg) for men or 50 pounds (22.5 kg) for women. Piked pushups involve elevating the feet or knees to simulate a handstand and performing a pushup from that position.

048

LEVEL I
For time:
3-mile (4.8 km) bike
30 goblet squats
10 inchworm pushups
5 wall walks

LEVEL II
For time:
4-mile (6.4 km) bike
40 goblet squats
15 inchworm pushups
10 wall walks

LEVEL III
For time:
5-mile (8 km) bike
50 goblet squats
25 inchworm pushups
10 wall walks

NOTES: Inchworm pushups should be done in place, walking the hands out to pushup position, then back to starting position after pushup. Goblet squats can be done with any object (kettlebell, dumbbell, etc.). Wall walks should be done to your ability level.

049

LEVEL I
3 rounds for time:
30 sledgehammer strikes
400-meter sledgehammer carry

LEVEL II
4 rounds for time:
30 sledgehammer strikes
400-meter sledgehammer carry

LEVEL III
5 rounds for time:
30 alternating sledgehammer strikes
400-meter sledgehammer carry

NOTES: Strikes should be performed on a tire, mound of dirt, etc. At level III, alternate arms after every strike. Sledgehammer strikes should be a downward movement from overhead with the sledge.

050

LEVEL I
EMOTM; 10-minutes:
:10 treading water
10 strokes freestyle

LEVEL II
EMOTM; 12-minutes:
:15 treading water
10 strokes freestyle

LEVEL III
EMOTM; 15-minutes:
:20 treading water
10 strokes freestyle

NOTES: This can be performed in a pool or open water where the feet can touch. At level III, athletes should tread water without the hands, if possible.

051

LEVEL I
3 rounds for completion:
10 rotating side planks
10 lateral lunges
10 seat rolls

LEVEL II
4 rounds for completion:
10 handstand shoulder touches against wall
10 lateral lunges
10 seat rolls

LEVEL III
5 rounds for completion:
10 freestanding handstand shoulder touches
10 lateral lunges
10 seat rolls

NOTES: This is a skill test with no time component. Focus should be on quality of repetitions, not speed. Side planks are performed on one elbow with the body facing the wall rather than the floor. Lateral lunges are sideways lunges.

052

LEVEL I
10-minute AMRAP:
5 air squats
10 hollow rocks
15 step ups

LEVEL II
15-minute AMRAP:
5 pistols
10 hollow rocks
15 box jumps

LEVEL III
20-minute AMRAP:
5 pistols
10 V ups
15 box jumps

NOTES: At level II, assist pistols by rolling or using a post. Ledges or stairs can be used as a substitute for boxes.

WODs AT HOME

053

LEVEL I
200-meter walking lunge with object
Every 25 steps perform 10 pushups

LEVEL II
300-meter walking lunge with object
Every 25 steps perform 10 hand release pushups

LEVEL III
400-meter walking lunge with object
Every 25 steps perform 10 hand release pushups

NOTES: Object may be any item 20 pounds (9 kg) or greater. Hands should be released at the bottom of the pushup movement to ensure the chest is on the ground.

054

LEVEL I
10 rounds for time:
5 burpees
5 sledgehammer strikes

LEVEL II
15 rounds for time:
5 burpees
5 sledgehammer strikes

LEVEL III
20 rounds for time:
5 burpees
5 sledgehammer strikes

NOTES: This is a high turnover workout, so transitions must be fasts. At level III, alternate sides for the strikes. Use a tire or mound of dirt for the sledgehammer strikes.

055

LEVEL I
100 burpee box jump overs for time

LEVEL II
100 burpee box jump overs for time

LEVEL III
100 burpee box jump overs for time

NOTES: Box can be any object or ledge 20 inches (51 cm) or higher.

056

LEVEL I
1-minute AMRAP burpees
2-minute rest
2-minute AMRAP burpees
4-minute rest
4-minute AMRAP burpees

LEVEL II
1-minute AMRAP burpees
1.5-minute rest
2-minute AMRAP burpees
3-minute rest
4-minute AMRAP burpees

LEVEL III
1-minute AMRAP burpees
1-minute rest
2-minute AMRAP burpees
2-minute rest
4-minute AMRAP burpees

NOTES: This is a pure conditioning test. The 1-minute set is a sprint, the 2-minute set is a semisprint, and the 4-minute set is moderate pace.

WODs AT HOME

057

LEVEL I
15-12-9 for time:
Step ups
Pushups
Situps

LEVEL II
21-15-9 for time:
Box jumps
Pushups
Situps

LEVEL III
21-15-9 for time:
Box jumps
Pushups
Situps

NOTE: Box jumps can be done on a ledge or step.

058

LEVEL I
For time:
1-mile (1.6 km) neighborhood run
10 wall walks
100 air squats

LEVEL II
For time:
1-mile (1.6 km) neighborhood run
50-meter handstand walk
Every fall complete 10 air squats

LEVEL III
For time:
1-mile (1.6 km) neighborhood run
100-meter handstand walk
Every fall complete 10 air squats

NOTES: Handstand walking is an approximate distance. If done outdoors, use gloves.

059

LEVEL I
3-×-400-meter sandbag sprint
Rest 3 minutes between efforts

LEVEL II
4-×-400-meter sandbag sprint
Rest 3 minutes between efforts

LEVEL III
5-×-400-meter sandbag sprint
Rest 3 minutes between efforts

NOTE: Sandbag can be carried in any fashion.

060

LEVEL I
12-minute AMRAP:
8 sandbag ground to shoulder
8 sandbag squats
8 sandbag shoulder to overhead
8 sandbag deadlifts

LEVEL II
15-minute AMRAP:
10 sandbag ground to shoulder
10 sandbag squats
10 sandbag shoulder to overhead
10 sandbag deadlifts

LEVEL III
20-minute AMRAP:
12 sandbag ground to shoulder
12 sandbag squats
12 sandbag shoulder to overhead
12 sandbag deadlifts

NOTE: Sandbag squats should be done with the bag on one shoulder or behind the neck.

WODs AT HOME

061

LEVEL I
6 rounds for time:
100-meter shuttle run
10 burpees

LEVEL II
8 rounds for time:
100-meter shuttle run
10 burpees

LEVEL III
10 rounds for time:
100-meter shuttle run
10 burpees

NOTES: Shuttle run should be 50 meters out and 50 meters back. This is meant to be done quickly.

062

LEVEL I
6 rounds for time:
10 squat jumps with rotation
50-meter swim

LEVEL II
8 rounds for time:
10 squat jumps with rotation
50-meter swim

LEVEL III
10 rounds for time:
10 squat jumps with rotation
50-meter swim

NOTES: If swimming pool is not available, substitute a run of 100 meters. The rotation on squat jumps should be 180 degrees, if possible.

063

LEVEL I
For time:
30-meter inchworm pushups
30-meter burpee broad jump
30-meter walking lunge
30-meter reverse walking lunge

LEVEL II
2 rounds for time:
30-meter inchworm pushups
30-meter burpee broad jump
30-meter walking lunge
30-meter reverse walking lunge

LEVEL III
3 rounds for time:
30-meter inchworm pushups
30-meter burpee broad jump
30-meter walking lunge
30-meter reverse walking lunge

NOTE: Each movement must be complete before moving on to the next.

064

LEVEL I
6 rounds for time at staircase:
Sprint up stairs
10 pushups

LEVEL II
8 rounds for time at staircase:
Sprint up stairs
20 pushups

LEVEL III
10 rounds for time at staircase:
Sprint up stairs
Bear crawl down stairs

NOTE: Staircase should be between 20 and 60 steps.

065

LEVEL I
100 sledgehammer strikes for completion

LEVEL II
100 sledgehammer strikes for completion

LEVEL III
100 sledgehammer strikes for completion

NOTE: At level II and level III, alternate sides after every strike.

066

LEVEL I
3 rounds for completion:
5 hollow rocks
5 air squats
5 hollow rocks
5 walking lunges
5 wall walks
5 forward rolls

LEVEL II
4 rounds for completion:
5 candlestick to deck squat
5 candlestick to pistol squat
5 wall handstands
5 forward rolls to stand
5 backward rolls to stand

LEVEL III
5 rounds for completion:
5 candlestick to deck squat
5 candlestick to pistol squat
5 handstand to forward roll
5 backward roll to handstand

NOTE: This should be done on soft carpet or grass with plenty of space around.

067

LEVEL I
10-minute AMRAP:
400-meter run
30 jumping jacks
15 pushups
10 good mornings

LEVEL II
15-minute AMRAP:
600-meter run
40 jumping jacks
20 pushups
10 good mornings

LEVEL III
20-minute AMRAP:
800-meter run
40 jumping jacks
20 pushups + lateral roll
10 weighted good mornings

NOTES: At level III, carry a weighted object during good mornings and alternate the direction of the lateral rolls with each repetition.

068

LEVEL I
21-15-9 for completion:
Pushups
Walking lunges
Back extensions

LEVEL II
21-15-9 for completion:
Piked pushup
Stationary lunges
Back extensions

LEVEL III
21-15-9 for completion:
Strict handstand pushup
Jumping lunges
Back extensions

NOTES: This is not for time, so don't rush through it. Back extensions should be performed from the prone position, arching the chest and shoulders as far away from the ground as possible during each repetition. "Strict" refers to the absence of any leg movement used to generate momentum.

069

LEVEL I
EMOTM; 10-minutes:
5 pushups
10 mountain climbers
50-meter sprint

LEVEL II
EMOTM; 12-minutes:
5 pushups
10 mountain climbers
75-meter sprint

LEVEL III
EMOTM; 15-minutes:
5 pushups
10 mountain climbers
100-meter sprint

NOTES: A mountain climber is completed when both knees have moved forward. Use time between rounds to rest and lower heart rate as much as possible.

070

LEVEL I
30 sandbag ground to overhead for time

LEVEL II
40 sandbag ground to overhead for time

LEVEL III
50 sandbag ground to overhead for time

NOTES: Sandbag can be filled to any weight. Any way from ground to overhead is acceptable, given good deadlift form off the ground.

071

LEVEL I
10-minute AMRAP:
5 jumping pullups
10 pushups
15 walking lunges

LEVEL II
15-minute AMRAP:
5 pullups
10 kick to handstand
15 jumping lunges

LEVEL III
20-minute AMRAP:
5 pullups
10 kick to handstand
15 jumping lunges

NOTES: Pullups can be performed on a tree branch, pullup bar, or any available object. Knee must touch ground on any lunge or jump lunge unless a preexisting injury prevents it.

072

LEVEL I
3 rounds for time:
3 sandbag thruster
6 sandbag lunge
9 sandbag hang clean

LEVEL II
4 rounds for time:
3 sandbag thruster
6 sandbag lunge
9 sandbag hang clean

LEVEL III
5 rounds for time:
3 sandbag thruster
6 sandbag lunge
9 sandbag hang clean

NOTES: Sandbag can be filled to any weight. For the lunges, sandbag should be thrown over one shoulder.

WODs AT HOME

073

LEVEL I
Sprint an increasing distance EMOTM; 10-minutes:
10-meters in minute 1
20-meters in minute 2
30-meters in minute 3
(and so forth)

LEVEL II
Sprint an increasing distance EMOTM; 10-minutes:
10-meters in minute 1
20-meters in minute 2
30-meters in minute 3
(and so forth)

LEVEL III
Sprint an increasing distance EMOTM; 10-minutes:
10-meters in minute 1
20-meters in minute 2
30-meters in minute 3
(and so forth)

NOTES: Sprints should be 90 percent effort unless the athlete is regularly practicing sprinting. *Do not* sprint 100 percent if you are not used to sprinting.

074

LEVEL I
For time:
100 single unders
60 squats
50 situps
40 pushups
30 squats
20 situps
10 pushups

LEVEL II
For time:
100 single unders
90 squats
80 situps
70 pushups
30 squats
20 situps
10 pushups

LEVEL III
For time:
100 single unders
90 squats
80 situps
70 pushups
60 squats
50 situps
40 pushups
30 squats
20 situps
10 pushups

NOTES: Situps should be done with straight legs. Pushups can be done from the knees for level I and level II, but must be from the toes for level III.

075

LEVEL I
10-minute AMRAP:
10-meter lateral bear crawl left
10 air squats
10-meter lateral bear crawl right

LEVEL II
12-minute AMRAP:
10-meter lateral wall walk left
10 deck squats
10-meter lateral wall walk right

LEVEL III
15-minute AMRAP:
10-meter lateral handstand walk left
10 deck squats
10-meter lateral handstand walk right

NOTES: At level II, attempt to wall walk in as close to a vertical handstand as possible. It is okay to resume a failed handstand walk from the point of failure.

076

LEVEL I
6 rounds for completion:
:30 butt kickers
5 burpees
:30 high knees
5 burpees

LEVEL II
8 rounds for completion:
:30 butt kickers
5 burpees
:30 high knees
5 burpees

LEVEL III
10 rounds for completion:
:30 butt kickers
5 burpees
:30 high knees
5 burpees

NOTE: Butt kickers and high knees should be done running in place.

077

LEVEL I
1-mile (1.6 km) neighborhood object carry
50 burpees for time

LEVEL II
1.5-mile (2.4 km) neighborhood object carry
75 burpees for time

LEVEL III
2-mile (3.2 km) neighborhood object carry
100 burpees for time

NOTES: Object can be anything over 20 pounds (9 kg). Burpees for time should be performed immediately upon return.

WODs AT HOME

078

LEVEL I
3 rounds for time:
10-meter lateral bear crawl left
10 pushups
10-meter lateral bear crawl right
10 pushups

LEVEL II
4 rounds for time:
20-meter lateral bear crawl left
10 pushups
20-meter lateral bear crawl right
10 pushups

LEVEL III
5 rounds for time:
20-meter lateral bear crawl left
10 clapping pushups
20-meter lateral bear crawl right
10 clapping pushups

NOTES: At level I and level II, do pushups from knees, but level III, they must be from toes.

079

LEVEL I
3 rounds for time:
20-meter broad jump
200-meter shuttle
Rest 1-minute between rounds

LEVEL II
4 rounds for time:
20-meter broad jump
200-meter shuttle
Rest 1-minute between rounds

LEVEL III
5 rounds for time:
20-meter broad jump
200-meter shuttle
Rest 1-minute between rounds

NOTE: Shuttle should be 100-meters out and 100-meters back.

080

LEVEL I
For time:
60 burpees to target
30 pushups
10 jumping pullups

LEVEL II
For time:
75 burpees to target
50 assisted ring dips
25 pullups

LEVEL III
For time:
90 burpees to target
60 ring dips
30 pullups

NOTES: Target should be set 6 inches (15 cm) above outstretched hand. Pullups can be done on any object in any manner. Ring dips can be assisted with a band or with the feet on the ground. Doing burpees to target means jumping and touching the hands to a target.

081

LEVEL I
50 deck squat burpees for time

LEVEL II
75 deck squat burpees for time

LEVEL III
100 deck squat burpees for time

NOTES: At level I and level II, use the hands to assist the deck squat; At level III may not. The deck squat portion of the movement is not complete until hips are fully extended. Only then can you begin the burpee.

082

LEVEL I
2-minute AMRAP:
10 pushups
10 hollow rocks
Rest 1-minute, repeat 3 rounds

LEVEL II
2-minute AMRAP:
10 pushups
:10 V sit hold
Rest 1-minute, repeat 4 rounds

LEVEL III
2-minute AMRAP:
10 pushups
:10 L sit hold
Rest 1-minute, repeat 5 rounds

NOTES: At level I and level II, do pushups from knees; At level IIImust be from toes. L sit holds can be done from the ground, paralettes, or boxes.

083

LEVEL I
3 rounds for time:
50-meter uphill lunges
50-meter downhill bear crawl

LEVEL II
4 rounds for time:
50-meter uphill lunges
50-meter downhill bear crawl

LEVEL III
5 rounds for time:
50-meter uphill lunges
50-meter downhill bear crawl

NOTES: The grade of the hill depends on the neighborhood. Pick the steepest one you can find and mark out the appropriate distance.

WODs AT HOME

084

LEVEL I
E2MOTM=Every two minutes "on the minute":
50-meter car push
10 pushups

LEVEL II
E2MOTM; 20-minutes:
75-meter car push
15 pushups

LEVEL III
E2MOTM; 20-minutes:
100-meter car push
20 pushups

NOTES: Find a flat stretch of road to avoid additional difficulty. Car push and pushups should be done as fast as possible to allow maximum rest time before the 2-minute interval is up.

085

LEVEL I
For time:
20 reverse burpees
20 sandbag front squats
20 pushups
800-meter run

LEVEL II
For time:
30 reverse burpees
30 sandbag front squats
30 piked pushups
800-meter run

LEVEL III
For time:
40 reverse burpees
40 sandbag front squats
40 handstand pushups
800-meter run

NOTES: Sandbag can be filled to any weight but must be held in front of the head, preferably with arms outstretched. Reverse burpees are performed by doing a deck squat and then a wall handstand. At level I and level II, use the hands to assist during deck squats.

086

LEVEL I
For completion:
Sandbag lunges 3-x-10
Sandbag press 3-x-10
Sandbag Carry-3-x-100-meters
Sandbag good mornings 3-x-10

LEVEL II
For completion:
Sandbag lunges 4-x-10
Sandbag press 4-x-10
Sandbag Carry-4-x-100-meters
Sandbag good mornings 4-x-10

LEVEL III
For completion:
Sandbag lunges 5-x-10
Sandbag press 5-x-10
Sandbag Carry-5-x-100-meters
Sandbag good mornings 5-x-10

NOTES: Sandbag can be filled to any weight. Exercises should be performed in alternating sequence, i.e., 10 lunges, 10 presses, 100-meters carry, 10 good mornings.

087

LEVEL I

For time:

30-meter lateral bear crawl right

Every 10 steps perform 20 mountain climbers, 10 pushups, 10 air squats

30-meter lateral bear crawl left

Every 10 steps perform 20 mountain climbers, 10 pushups, 10 air squats

LEVEL II

For time:

40-meter lateral bear crawl right

Every 10 steps perform 20 mountain climbers, 10 pushups, 10 air squats

40-meter lateral bear crawl left

Every 10 steps perform 20 mountain climbers, 10 pushups, 10 air squats

LEVEL III

For time:

50-meter lateral bear crawl right

Every 10 steps perform 20 mountain climbers, 10 pushups, 10 air squats

50-meter lateral bear crawl left

Every 10 steps perform 20 mountain climbers, 10 pushups, 10 air squats

NOTES: Every movement with the lead hand counts as a step. The mountain climbers, pushups, and air squats should be completed in unbroken sets for level III. Level I, may do pushups from the knees.

088

LEVEL I

6-minute AMRAP:

10 single arm object swings right

10-meter waiter's walk right

10 single arm object swings left

10-meter waiter's walk left

LEVEL II

8-minute AMRAP:

10 single arm object swings right

10-meter waiter's walk right

10 single arm object swings left

10-meter waiter's walk left

LEVEL III

10-minute AMRAP:

10 single arm object swings right

10-meter waiter's walk right

10 single arm object swings left

10-meter waiter's walk left

NOTES: Object can be a kettlebell, dumbbell, paint can, etc. Single arm swings should be Russian style (eye level); waiter's walk is simulating a waiter holding a tray overhead and should be fully locked out.

WODs AT HOME

089

LEVEL I
3 rounds for time:
400-meter run
30 air squats
20 pushups
10 situps

LEVEL II
4 rounds for time:
800-meter run
40 air squats
30 pushups
20 situps

LEVEL III
5 rounds for time:
800-meter run
50 air squats
40 pushups
30 situps

NOTES: This is intended to be paced steadily, so do not go out too fast. At level I, do pushups from the knees if necessary. Situps should be done with straight legs.

090

LEVEL I
8-minute AMRAP:
10-meter duck walk
5 wall walks
10-meter frog hop
10-meter bear crawl

LEVEL II
10-minute AMRAP:
10-meter duck walk
7 wall walks
10-meter frog hop
10-meter low crawl

LEVEL III
12-minute AMRAP:
10-meter duck walk
10-meter handstand walk
10-meter frog hop
10-meter low crawl

NOTES: Use a 10-meter space of carpet, matting, or grass. Duck walk is walk while in a low squat. Low crawl should be on knees and elbows. Frog hop is hopping from low squat to low squat.

091

LEVEL I
E2MOTM; 20-minutes:
5 situps
10 pushups
15 air squats
100-meter run

LEVEL II
E2MOTM; 30-minutes:
5 situps
10 pushups
15 air squats
200-meter run

LEVEL III
E2MOTM; 40-minutes:
5 situps
10 pushups
15 air squats
300-meter run

NOTES: Complete one round of the workout every 2 minutes until failure to complete. Upon failure to complete the round in 2 minutes, the workout is over.

092

LEVEL I
3 rounds:
30 burpees for time
Rest exactly the time taken to complete.

LEVEL II
3 rounds:
40 burpees for time
Rest exactly the time taken to complete.

LEVEL III
3 rounds:
50 burpees for time
Rest exactly the time taken to complete.

NOTES: These efforts should be sprints for all levels. The goal is to improve the speed of the movement at high heart rates.

093

LEVEL I
EMOTM; 12-minutes:
20-meter bear crawl shuttle

LEVEL II
EMOTM; 16-minutes:
30-meter bear crawl shuttle

LEVEL III
EMOTM; 20-minutes:
30-meter bear crawl shuttle

NOTES: Every minute, must complete a down and back bear crawl totaling the prescribed distance. The faster the distance is completed, the more rest you get.

094

LEVEL I
200-meter sandbag carry for time
Every 20 steps complete 5 sandbag squats

LEVEL II
300-meter sandbag carry for time
Every 20 steps complete 5 sandbag squats

LEVEL III
400-meter sandbag carry for time
Every 20 steps complete 5 sandbag squats

NOTE: Sandbag should be filled to a weight where athletes can complete 5 squats comfortably.

095

LEVEL I
3 rounds for time:
25-meter car push out
25-meter car push back
20 sandbag deadlifts
5 wall walks

LEVEL II
4 rounds for time:
25-meter car push out
25-meter car push back
20 sandbag deadlifts
5 handstand pushups

LEVEL III
5 rounds for time:
25-meter car push out
25-meter car push back
20 sandbag deadlifts
10 handstand pushups

NOTES: Sandbags can be filled to any weight. Handstand pushups should be done with a mat or shirt under head.

096

LEVEL I
Perform an additional sledgehammer strike EMOTM until failure to complete in prescribed minute.
1 strike in minute 1
2 strikes in minute 2
3 strikes in minute 3
(and so forth)

LEVEL II
Perform an additional sledgehammer strike EMOTM until failure to complete in prescribed minute.
1 strike in minute 1
2 strikes in minute 2
3 strikes in minute 3
(and so forth)

LEVEL III
Perform an additional sledgehammer strike EMOTM until failure to complete in prescribed minute.
1 strike in minute 1
2 strikes in minute 2
3 strikes in minute 3
(and so forth)

NOTES: Strike a tire or mound of dirt with the sledge. At level III, alternate sides for each swing.

WODs AT HOME

097

LEVEL I
10-minute AMRAP:
100-meter shuttle run
5 burpees

LEVEL II
10-minute AMRAP:
100-meter shuttle run
5 burpees

LEVEL III
10-minute AMRAP:
100-meter shuttle run
5 burpees

NOTES: No need to scale this workout. All levels should be able to complete as written.

098

LEVEL I
100 single unders for time
EMOTM complete 5 sandbag ground to shoulder

LEVEL II
250 double unders for time
EMOTM complete 5 sandbag ground to shoulder

LEVEL III
500 double unders for time
EMOTM complete 5 sandbag ground to shoulder

NOTE: Sandbags can be filled to any weight.

099

LEVEL I
3 rounds for time:
10 superman rocks
10 deck squats
10 pushups
Rest 2 minutes and repeat

LEVEL II
5 rounds for time:
10 superman rocks
10 deck squats
10 pushups
Rest 2 minutes and repeat

LEVEL III
5 rounds for time:
10 superman rocks
10 deck squats
10 clapping pushups
Rest 2 minutes and repeat

NOTES: At level I and level II, do pushups from knees and use hands during deck squats. Level III, may not.

100

LEVEL I
21-15-9
Sandbag thrusters
Jumping pullups

LEVEL II
21-15-9
Sandbag thrusters
Pullups

LEVEL III
21-15-9
Sandbag thrusters
Pullups

NOTES: Pullups can be done on any object, such as a tree branch or decking. Sandbags can be filled to any weight.

101

LEVEL I
5 rounds for time:
20 step ups
20 burpees
20 bicycle crunches
10 hip bridges

LEVEL II
5 rounds for time:
20 box jumps
20 man on fire burpees
20 bicycle crunches
10 hip bridges

LEVEL III
5 rounds for time:
20 box jumps
20 man on fire burpees
20 V ups
10 full bridges

NOTES: Box jumps and step ups can be done on any object (stair, step, wall, etc). Man on fire burpees are performed by laterally rolling between burpees.

WODs AT HOME

102

LEVEL I
For time:
50-meter broad jump
15 pushups
50-meter broad jump
15 situps
50-meter broad jump
15 pushups
50-meter broad jump

LEVEL II
For time:
75-meter broad jump
20 pushups
75-meter broad jump
20 situps
75-meter broad jump
20 bench dips
75-meter broad jump

LEVEL III
For time:
100-meter broad jump
25 pushups
100-meter broad jump
25 situps
100-meter broad jump
25 bench dips
100-meter broad jump

NOTES: Reset between each broad jump rather than bounding between. At level I and level II, do pushups from knees. Bench dips can be done on any ledge.

103

LEVEL I
Accumulate 1-minute in a headstand
Accumulate 1-minute in an L sit
Accumulate 1-minute in a plank
Accumulate 1-minute in side plank
Accumulate 1-minute in a handstand

LEVEL II
Accumulate 2 minutes in a headstand
Accumulate 2 minutes in an L sit
Accumulate 2 minutes in a plank
Accumulate 2 minutes in side plank
Accumulate 2 minutes in a handstand

LEVEL III
Accumulate 3 minutes in a headstand
Accumulate 3 minutes in an L sit
Accumulate 3 minutes in a plank
Accumulate 3 minutes in side plank
Accumulate 3 minutes in a handstand

NOTES: Find a soft area to practice these skills. L sits can be done from support or hanging. Side planks should be alternated every 30 seconds.

104

LEVEL I
Perform 6 pushups, then push wheelbarrow the prescribed distance EMOTM until failure to complete:

10-meters

20-meters

30-meters

(and so forth)

LEVEL II
Perform 8 pushups, then push wheelbarrow the prescribed distance EMOTM until failure to complete:

10-meters

20-meters

30-meters

(and so forth)

LEVEL III
Perform 10 pushups, then push wheelbarrow the prescribed distance EMOTM until failure to complete:

10-meters

20-meters

30-meters

(and so forth)

NOTES: The pushups are the prerequisite for every round. The remaining time is to be used to push the wheelbarrow the required distance and then rest for the next round. Wheelbarrow can be loaded to any weight.

105

LEVEL I
50 sandbag squats for time
EMOTM complete 5 shoulder to overhead

LEVEL II
75 sandbag squats for time
EMOTM complete 5 shoulder to overhead

LEVEL III
100 sandbag squats for time
EMOTM complete 5 shoulder to overhead

NOTES: Sandbags should be loaded on back or shoulders. They can be filled to any weight. Shoulder to overhead can be completed in any fashion.

106

LEVEL I
3 rounds for completion:
5 sandbag push press
10 sandbag bent row
15 sandbag front squat

LEVEL II
4 rounds for completion:
5 sandbag push press
10 sandbag bent row
15 sandbag front squat

LEVEL III
5 rounds for completion:
5 sandbag push press
10 sandbag bent row
15 sandbag front squat

NOTES: Sandbags can be loaded to any weight. Bent rows should be performed with torso parallel to the ground and knees slightly bent.

107

LEVEL I
10-minute AMRAP:
10 lateral hurdle hops
10 seat rolls
10 lunges
10-meter inchworm walk

LEVEL II
15-minute AMRAP:
15 lateral hurdle hops
15 seat rolls
15 jump lunges
15-meter inchworm walk

LEVEL III
20-minute AMRAP:
20 lateral hurdle hops
20 seat rolls
20 jump lunges
20-meter handstand walk

NOTES: Hurdle hops can be over imaginary hurdle if necessary, but are intended to be sideways jumps. Seat rolls begin and end on seat, passing through the top of pushup position. Inchworm walk is done with straight legs, walking hands out to full body extension and then walking feet forward to hands.

108

LEVEL I

For time:

Every 5 yards (4.5 m) for 100 yards (91.5 m), complete 5 burpees

Every 5 yards (4.5 m) for 100 yards (91.5 m), complete 5 lunges

Every 5 yards (4.5 m) for 100 yards (91.5 m), complete 5 pushups

Every (4.5 m) for 100 yards (91.5 m), complete 5 air squats

LEVEL II

For time:

Every 5 yards (4.5 m) for 100 yards (91.5 m), complete 5 burpees

Every 5 yards (4.5 m) for 100 yards (91.5 m), complete 5 jump lunges

Every 5 yards (4.5 m) for 100 yards (91.5 m), complete 5 pushups

Every 5 yards (4.5 m) for 100 yards (91.5 m), complete 5 deck squats

LEVEL III

For time:

Every 5 yards (4.5 m) for 100 yards (91.5 m), complete 5 burpees

Every 5 yards (4.5 m) for 100 yards (91.5 m), complete 5 jump lunges

Every 5 yards (4.5 m) for 100 yards (91.5 m), complete 5 clapping pushups

Every 5 yards (4.5 m) for 100 yards (91.5 m), complete 5 deck squats

NOTES: For this workout, find a school or park that has a football field or soccer pitch.

109

LEVEL I

6-x-40-meter dash
Rest 2 minutes between efforts
3-x-max pushups
Rest 2 minutes between efforts

LEVEL II

8-x-40-meter dash
Rest 2 minutes between efforts
4-x-max pushups
Rest 2 minutes between efforts

LEVEL III

10-x-40-meter dash
Rest 2 minutes between efforts
5-x-max pushups
Rest 2 minutes between efforts

NOTES: For this workout, find a school or park that has a football field or soccer pitch. All 40-meter dashes should be finished before begining max effort pushups.

WODs AT HOME

110

LEVEL I
For time:
6 to 1 sandbag clean and jerk
50-meter sandbag carry

LEVEL II
For time:
8 to 1 sandbag clean and jerk
50-meter sandbag carry

LEVEL III
For time:
10 to 1 sandbag clean and jerk
50-meter sandbag carry

NOTES: Sandbag can be filled to any weight. "6 to 1" means 6, 5, 4, 3, 2, 1 repetitions.

111

LEVEL I
10-minute AMRAP:
Odd minutes complete AMRAP object squats
Even minutes run 200-meters

LEVEL II
15-minute AMRAP:
Odd minutes complete AMRAP object squats
Even minutes run 200-meters

LEVEL III
20-minute AMRAP:
Odd minutes complete AMRAP object squats
Even minutes run 200-meters

NOTES: Object can be anything over 50 pounds (22.5 kg) for men or over 30 pounds (13.5 kg) for women. Objects can be squatted in any manner. Score for the workout is total number of squats.

112

LEVEL I
EMOTM; 10-minutes:
1 wall walk
3 burpees
5 step ups

LEVEL II
EMOTM; 15-minutes:
2 wall walks
4 burpees
6 box jumps

LEVEL III
EMOTM; 20-minutes:
3 wall walks
5 burpees
7 box jumps

NOTES: Wall walks should be done to ability level, meaning get as close to the wall as capable of safely. At level III, touch your chest to the wall. Ledges or stairs can be used for box jumps and step ups.

113

LEVEL I
For completion:
30 percent bodyweight carry up 400-meter hill

LEVEL II
2 rounds for completion:
30 percent bodyweight carry up 400-meter hill

LEVEL III
3 rounds for completion:
30 percent bodyweight carry up 400-meter hill

NOTES: You can use sandbags to complete workout, but do not have to. Any object that is 30 percent bodyweight will suffice.

114

LEVEL I
20-10-5 for time:
Sandbag snatch
Burpees over sandbag
Single unders

LEVEL II
20-15-10 for time:
Sandbag snatch
Burpees over sandbag
Double unders

LEVEL III
30-20-10 for time:
Sandbag snatch
Burpees over sandbag
Double unders

NOTES: Sandbag can be filled to any weight. Burpees should include a 2-foot (61 cm) jump over a sandbag.

WODs AT HOME

115

LEVEL I
For time:
100-meter walking lunge
300-meter run
100-meter bear crawl
300-meter run
100-meter crab walk
300-meter run
100-meter broad jump
300-meter run

LEVEL II
For time:
100-meter walking lunge
300-meter run
100-meter bear crawl
300-meter run
100-meter crab walk
300-meter run
100-meter broad jump
300-meter run

LEVEL III
For time:
100-meter walking lunge
300-meter run
100-meter bear crawl
300-meter run
100-meter crab walk
300-meter run
100-meter broad jump
300-meter run

NOTES: Find a park, school, or track to complete this workout. Pace should be slow and steady on the 100-meter efforts. Focus on striding out the 300-meter runs.

116

LEVEL I
3 rounds for time:
:30 high knees
50-meter sprint
10 burpees
50-meter sprint
10 sandbag thrusters
50-meter sprint

LEVEL II
4 rounds for time:
:30 high knees
75-meter sprint
10 burpees
75-meter sprint
10 sandbag thrusters
75-meter sprint

LEVEL III
5 rounds for time:
:30 high knees
100-meter sprint
10 burpees
100-meter sprint
10 sandbag thrusters
100-meter sprint

NOTES: This is a sprint-style workout. Burpees and thrusters should be done unbroken and as quickly as possible. Sandbag can be filled to any weight.

117

LEVEL I
100-meter bear crawl
Every 10-meters complete
10 situps
10 air squats

LEVEL II
50-meter handstand walk
Every 10-meters complete
10 situps
10 deck squats

LEVEL III
100-meter handstand walk
Every 10-meters complete
15 situps
15 deck squats

NOTES: The situps and squats are the built-in breaks for this workout. Handstand walking should be under control and steady.

118

LEVEL I
2-minute AMRAP:
1 ring pullup
2 hand release pushups
3 box jumps
Rest 1-minute, complete 3 rounds

LEVEL II
2-minute AMRAP:
1 muscle up
2 piked pushups
3 box jumps
Rest 1-minute, complete 4 rounds

LEVEL III
2-minute AMRAP:
1 muscle up
2 strict handstand pushups
3 box jumps
Rest 1-minute, complete 5 rounds

NOTES: This is a sprint, so move quickly between exercises. At level II, kip the handstand pushups if necessary. Stairs and ledges can be used for box jumps.

119

LEVEL I
For time:
10-meter shuttle
20-meter shuttle
30-meter shuttle
40-meter shuttle
50-meter shuttle
60-meter shuttle

LEVEL II
For time:
10-meter shuttle
20-meter shuttle
30-meter shuttle
40-meter shuttle
50-meter shuttle
60-meter shuttle
70-meter shuttle
80-meter shuttle

LEVEL III
For time:
10-meter shuttle
20-meter shuttle
30-meter shuttle
40-meter shuttle
50-meter shuttle
60-meter shuttle
70-meter shuttle
80-meter shuttle
90-meter shuttle
100-meter shuttle

NOTES: This is a pure conditioning test. Find a football field or track with markers for this workout. The 10-meter shuttle is 5-meters out and 5 back; the 20-meter shuttle is 10-meters out, 10 back, etc.

120

LEVEL I
1-minute sandbag carry for max distance
Rest 1 minute
2-minute sandbag carry for max distance
Rest 2 minutes
4-minute sandbag carry for max distance

LEVEL II
1-minute sandbag carry for max distance
Rest 1 minute
2-minute sandbag carry for max distance
Rest 2 minutes
4-minute sandbag carry for max distance

LEVEL III
1-minute sandbag carry for max distance
Rest 1 minute
2-minute sandbag carry for max distance
Rest 2 minutes
4-minute sandbag carry for max distance

NOTES: Score for this workout is total distance traveled. Sandbag can be loaded to any weight.

121

LEVEL I
2 rounds for time:
50-meter suitcase carry left arm
50-meter suitcase carry right arm
50-meter waiter's walk left arm
50-meter waiter's walk right arm
10 push press left arm
10 push press right arm

LEVEL II
2 rounds for time:
75-meter suitcase carry left arm
75-meter suitcase carry right arm
75-meter waiter's walk left arm
75-meter waiter's walk right arm
10 push press left arm
10 push press right arm

LEVEL III
3 rounds for time:
100-meter suitcase carry left arm
100-meter suitcase carry right arm
100-meter waiter's walk left arm
100-meter waiter's walk right arm
10 push press left arm
10 push press right arm

NOTES: The same object, such as a kettlebell, dumbbell, paint can, etc, should be used for all movements. Any weight will work for all levels. Suitcase carry is a walk with one arm and weight by side. Waiter's walk is with one arm and weight overhead.

122

LEVEL I
E5MOTM; 20-minutes:
20-meter lateral shuffle
80-meter sprint
20 pushups

LEVEL II
E4MOTM; 20-minutes:
20-meter lateral shuffle
80-meter sprint
20 pushups

LEVEL III
E2MOTM; 20-minutes:
20-meter lateral shuffle
80-meter sprint
20 pushups

NOTES: At level I, perform 1 round of the workout every 5 minutes. At level II, perform 1 round of the workout every 4 minutes. At level III, perform 1 round of the workout every 2 minutes. Lateral shuffle should alternate directions each round.

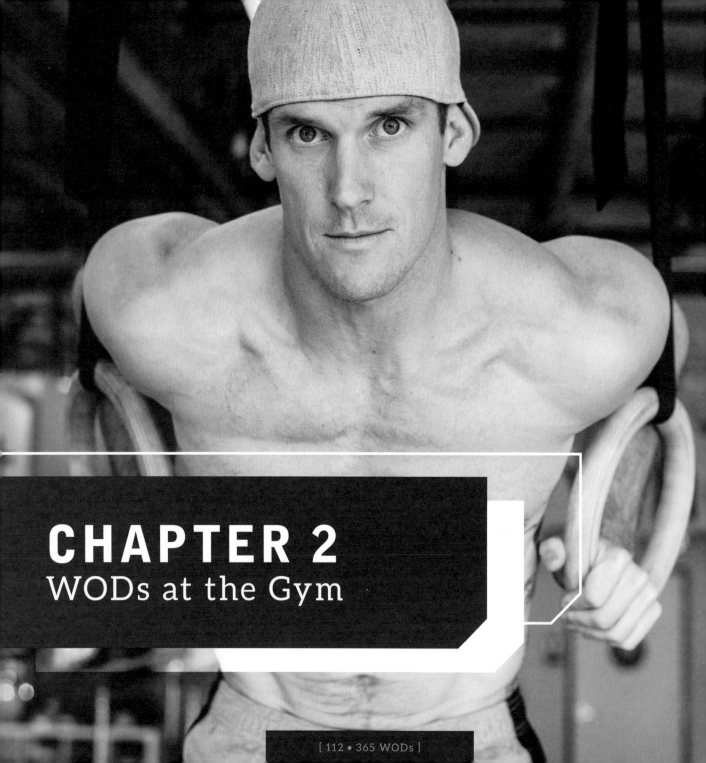

CHAPTER 2
WODs at the Gym

This section is written for readers who can train with a CrossFit box or in another functional fitness facility. Many of the workouts include lifts that will require Olympic barbells and bumper plates, climbing ropes, kettlebells, medicine balls, and more. This is not to say that the workouts can't be adapted to a more traditional gym setting, only that precautions must be taken with the equipment when doing so. At level I, you will need to be patient and spend most of the early workouts practicing technique on the more difficult lifts. It will not benefit you to rush into a level II or level III workout until you have learned to do all the moves safely.

WODs AT THE GYM

123

LEVEL I
21-15-9
Push ups
Bent leg situps

LEVEL II
21-15-9
Push press (95 pounds [43 kg]/65 pounds [29.5 kg])
Straight leg situps

LEVEL III
21-15-9
Push press (135 pounds [61 kg]/95 pounds [43 kg])
Toes to bar

NOTES: This is a sprint-style workout. Attempt to do as much of it unbroken as possible.

95 pounds (43 kg)/65 pounds (29.5 kg) = This notation refers to lift weight for men and women, respectively.

124

LEVEL I
10-minute AMRAP:
50-meter sled drag
10 ring rows
10 burpees

LEVEL II
15-minute AMRAP:
50-meter sled drag
10 pullups
20 burpees

LEVEL III
15-minute AMRAP:
50-meter sled drag
5 muscle ups
20 burpees

NOTES: The weight of the sled is up to you.

125

LEVEL I

8 Tabata intervals:
Airdyne for distance
Pushups
Single unders
Row for calories

LEVEL II

8 Tabata intervals:
Airdyne for distance
Hand release pushups
Double unders
Row for calories

LEVEL III

8 Tabata intervals:
Airdyne for distance
Hand release pushups
Double unders
Row for calories

NOTES: Tabata means that you should give 80 percent effort or higher for 20 seconds, then rest for 10 seconds. After eight intervals of one exercise, move to the next without resting.

126

LEVEL I

20-15-10
Ball slam
Ring rows

LEVEL II

30-20-10
Wall ball
Pullups

LEVEL III

30-20-10
Wall ball
Chest to bar pullups

NOTES: Use a 20-pound (9 kg) medicine ball for men, 14-pound (6.5 kg) medicine ball for women. Men aim for a 10-foot (3 m) target; women aim for a 9-foot (2.7 m) target.

WODs AT THE GYM

127

LEVEL I
For time:
500-meter row
30 single arm dumbbell swings
25-meter burpee broad jump

LEVEL II
For time:
750-meter row
30 dumbbell ground to overhead
25-meter burpee broad jump

LEVEL III
For time:
1000-meter row
50 dumbbell ground to overhead
25-meter burpee broad jump

NOTES: At level I, do Russian-style swings (eye level). At level II and level III, touch the dumbbell to the ground between repetitions. You may alternate arms whenever you choose.

128

LEVEL I
4 rounds for time:
20 bodyweight walking lunges
200-meter run
20-meter bear crawl

LEVEL II
4 rounds for time:
20 barbell walking lunges (45 pounds [20.5 kg]/35 pounds [16 kg])
100-meter barbell carry (45 pounds [20.5 kg]/35 pounds [16 kg])
10-meter handstand walk

LEVEL III
5 rounds for time:
20 barbell walking lunges (95 pounds [43 kg]/65 pounds [29.5 kg])
100-meter barbell carry (45 pounds [20.5 kg]/35 pounds [16 kg])
20-meter handstand walk

NOTES: Barbell should be on the back for walking lunges and barbell carry. Handstand walk does not need to be completed unbroken.

129

LEVEL I

3 rounds for time:
7 jumping pullups
7 pushups
21 kettlebell swings (35 pounds [16 kg]/25 pounds [11.5 kg])

LEVEL II

3 rounds for time:
3 muscle ups
21 kettlebell swings (55 pounds [25 kg]/35 pounds [16 kg])

LEVEL III

3 rounds for time:
7 muscle ups
21 kettlebell swings (70 pounds [32 kg]/50 pounds [22.5 kg])

NOTE: At level I, do Russian-style swings (eye level); At level II and level III, do American-style swings (overhead). All levels should do as much of the workout unbroken as possible.

130

LEVEL I

Back squat 3-x-5
Conventional deadlift 3-x-5
Good morning 4-x-8
Situp 4-x-8

LEVEL II

Back squat 3-x-3
Conventional deadlift 7-x-1
Back extension 4-x-8
Toes to bar 4-x-8

LEVEL III

Box squat 3-x-3
Conventional deadlift 10-x-1
Glute ham raise 4-x-8
Strict toes to bar 4-x-8

NOTES: All weights are determined by the strength of the individual. The goal is to find the heaviest weight possible for the prescribed number of repetitions. However, do not sacrifice technique for load. Glute ham raise is when the athlete follows a back extension is followed with a leg curl.

WODs AT THE GYM

131

LEVEL I
Floor press 4-x-5
Rope climb to standing 5-x-3
Abmat situp 3-x-25
Dead hang 3-x-max

LEVEL II
Floor press 7-x-3
Rope climb 5-x-1
Abmat situp 3-x-25
Strict pullup 2-x-max

LEVEL III
Floor press 10-x-3
Rope climb 5-x-1
GHD situp 3-x-25
Strict pullup 3-x-max

NOTES: All weights are determined by the strength of the individual. The goal is to find the heaviest weight possible for the prescribed number of repetitions. However, do not sacrifice technique for load. If athletes do not know how to climb rope using a foot lock, use this section as practice.

132

LEVEL I
Hang power snatch 5-x-1
Clean and Jerk technique 10 minutes practice
Front squat 3-x-5

LEVEL II
Hang power snatch 5-x-1
2 cleans + 1 jerk-x-5
Front squat 4-x-3

LEVEL III
Hang power snatch 5-x-1
2 cleans + 1 jerk-x-5
Front squat 4-x-3

NOTES: All weights are determined by the strength of the individual. The goal is to find the heaviest weight possible for the prescribed number of repetitions. However, do not sacrifice technique for load.

133

LEVEL I
Snatch 5-x-3
Hang clean and jerk 10 minutes practice
Front squat 3-x-5

LEVEL II
1 snatch EMOTM 10 minutes at 75 percent 1RM
Hang clean and jerk + 20 second overhead hold-x-3
Front squat 4-x-4

LEVEL III
2 snatch EMOTM 10 minutes at 85 percent 1RM
Hang clean and jerk + 20 second overhead hold-x-5
Front squat 4-x-4

NOTES: If you don't know your percentages, work up to a difficult weight and operate there. Overhead holds should be static. 1RM stands for one repetition maximum.

134

LEVEL I
Barbell strict press 5-x-5
Bent row 5-x-8
Situp 3-x-20
Ring row 3-x-max reps

LEVEL II
Barbell strict press 7-x-2
Bent row 4-x-5
Strict knee to elbow 3-x-max reps
Strict chinup 3-x-max reps

LEVEL III
Barbell strict press 10-x-2
Bent row 5-x-5
Strict toes to bar 3-x-max reps
Strict chinup 3-x-max reps

NOTES: All weights are determined by the strength of the individual. The goal is to find the heaviest weight possible for the prescribed number of repetitions. However, do not sacrifice technique for load.

WODs AT THE GYM

135

LEVEL I
Back squat 5-x-1
Deadlift 5-x-5
Good morning 3-x-10
400-meter sled drag

LEVEL II
Establish 1RM back squat
Deadlift 7-x-2
Glute ham raise 3-x-8
400-meter heavy sled drag

LEVEL III
Establish 1RM back squat
Deadlift 10-x-2
Glute ham raise 4-x-8
400-meter heavy sled drag

NOTES: All weights are determined by the strength of the individual. The goal is to find the heaviest weight possible for the prescribed number of repetitions. However, do not sacrifice technique for load. At level I, may use empty sled. At level II and level III, load the sled to a heavy weight.

136

LEVEL I
Floor press 5-x-3
Assisted chinup 5-x-5
Pushup 3-x-10
Hollow rock 3-x-20

LEVEL II
Floor press 7-x-3
Chinup 7-x-7
Bar dip 3-x-10
Hollow rock 3-x-30

LEVEL III
Floor press 10-x-3
Weighted chinup 10-x-1
Ring dip 3-x-10
Hollow rock 3-x-40

NOTES: All weights are determined by the strength of the individual. The goal is to find the heaviest weight possible for the prescribed number of repetitions. However, do not sacrifice technique for load. At level I, assist chinups using a band or a box.

137

LEVEL I
10 to 1 ring rows
1 to 10 kettlebell swings

LEVEL II
10 to 1 pullups
1 to 10 kettlebell snatch each arm

LEVEL III
10 to 1 muscle ups
1 to 10 kettlebell snatch each arm

NOTES: At level I, do American-style swings (overhead). At level II and level III, alternate arms every rep for kettlebell snatch. 10 to 1 refers to a descending repetition scheme from 10 down to 1.

138

LEVEL I
Back squat 3-x-3
Overhead squat 10 minutes practice
Sumo deadlift 4-x-5
Good morning 3-x-8

LEVEL II
Back squat 5-x-3
Overhead squat 3-x-10
Sumo deadlift 4-x-5
Good morning 3-x-8

LEVEL III
Back squat 7-x-3
Overhead squat 5-x-5
Sumo deadlift 6-x-5
Weighted good morning 3-x-8

NOTES: All weights are determined by the strength of the individual. The goal is to find the heaviest weight possible for the prescribed number of repetitions. However, do not sacrifice technique for load.

139

LEVEL I
Bench press 5-x-5
Ring row 3-x-10
Rope climb to standing 3-x-3

LEVEL II
Bench press 7-x-2
Chinup 5-x-5
Rope climb 3-x-1

LEVEL III
Bench press with chains 10-x-2
Weighted chinup with chains 5-x-5
Rope climb 3-x-3

NOTES: All weights are determined by the strength of the individual. The goal is to find the heaviest weight possible for the prescribed number of repetitions. However, do not sacrifice technique for load. If chains ar e unavailable, complete lifts without them.

WODs AT THE GYM

140

LEVEL I
Box squat 5-x-3
Conventional deadlift 5-x-5
Back extension 3-x-8
Ring row 3-x-10

LEVEL II
Box squat 7-x-1
Conventional deadlift 7-x-1
Back extension 4-x-8
Bent row 3-x-8

LEVEL III
Box squat 10-x-1
Conventional deadlift with bands 10-x-1
Glute ham raise 4-x-8
Bent row 3-x-8

NOTES: All weights are determined by the strength of the individual. The goal is to find the heaviest weight possible for the prescribed number of repetitions. However, do not sacrifice technique for load.

141

LEVEL I
30 clean and jerks for time (95 pounds [43 kg]/65 pounds [29.5 kg])

LEVEL II
30 clean and jerks for time (115 pounds [52 kg]/75 pounds [34 kg])

LEVEL III
30 clean and jerks for time (135 pounds [61 kg]/95 pounds [43 kg])

NOTES: This is a sprint-style workout. At level I, attempt to make every rep perfect; At level II and level III, focus on speed.

142

LEVEL I
Barbell strict press 3 reps EMOTM 10 minutes
Bent row 3-x-5
Wall walk 3-x-5
Ring row 3-x-10

LEVEL II
Barbell strict press 3 reps EMOTM 10 minutes
Bent row 4-x-5
Handstand hold against wall 3-x-max time
Ring pullup 3-x-10

LEVEL III
Barbell strict press 3 reps EMOTM 10 minutes
Bent row 6-x-5
Strict handstand pushup 3-x-max
Ring pullup 3-x-10

NOTES: All weights are determined by the strength of the individual. The goal is to find the heaviest weight possible for the prescribed number of repetitions. However, do not sacrifice technique for load.

143

LEVEL I

Snatch 10 minutes practice
Hang power clean and jerk 5-x-2
Front squat 3-x-5

LEVEL II

1 snatch EMOTM; 10 minutes at
80 percent 1RM
Hang squat clean and jerk 7-x-2
Front squat 4-x-5

LEVEL III

1 snatch EMOTM; 10 minutes at
90 percent 1RM
Hang squat clean and jerk 10-x-2
Front squat 5-x-5

NOTES: If athletes don't know their
percentages, they should work up to
a heavy single and operate there for
the snatches. The other weights are
determined by the strength of the lifter.

144

LEVEL I

Walking lunge 3-x-10 each leg
Pushup 3-x-10
GHD situp 3-x-20
Rope climb to standing 5-x-3

LEVEL II

Weighted lunge 5-x-5 each leg
Kneeling strict press 4-x-5
Abmat situp 3-x-20
Rope climb 5-x-1

LEVEL III

Weighted lunge 5-x-5 each leg
Kneeling strict press 5-x-5
GHD situp 3-x-20
Legless rope climb 5-x-1

NOTES: All weights are determined
by the strength of the individual. The
goal is to find the heaviest weight
possible for the prescribed number of
repetitions. However, do not sacrifice
technique for load.

145

LEVEL I

3 rounds for time:
400-meter run
9 kettlebell swings (35 pounds
[16 kg]/25 pounds [11.5 kg])
9 hang cleans (95 pounds
[43 kg]/65 pounds [29.5 kg])

LEVEL II

3 rounds for time:
400-meter run
15 kettlebell swings (55 pounds
[25 kg]/35 pounds [16 kg])
15 hang cleans (135 pounds
[61 kg]/95 pounds [43 kg])

LEVEL III

3 rounds for time:
400-meter run
21 kettlebell swings (55 pounds
[25 kg]/35 pounds [16 kg])
21 hang cleans (185 pounds
[84 kg]/115 pounds [52 kg])

NOTES: Weights are intended to
be heavy for the hang cleans so
you will need to break up the sets
strategically. Time will be made up
on the runs and kettlebell swings.
At level I, do Russian-style swings
(eye level). At level II and level III, do
American-style swings (overhead).

WODs AT THE GYM

146

LEVEL I
Barbell push press + 5 second eccentric 5-x-2
Dumbbell row 3-x-5
Wall walk 3-x-5

LEVEL II
Barbell push press + 5 second eccentric 7-x-2
Dumbbell row 4-x-5
Wall walk 3-x-7

LEVEL III
Barbell push press + 5 second eccentric 10-x-2
Dumbbell row 5-x-5
Wall walk 3-x-10

NOTES: All weights are determined by the strength of the individual. The goal is to find the heaviest weight possible for the prescribed number of repetitions. However, do not sacrifice technique for load. "Eccentric" refers to the lowering of the bar to the chest.

147

LEVEL I
1-mile (1.6 km) Airdyne sprint for time

LEVEL II
1-mile (1.6 km) Airdyne sprint for time

LEVEL III
1-mile (1.6 km) Airdyne sprint for time

NOTES: This is an all-out sprint. Do not hold back. Upon completion, stay on the bike and ride an easy 3-miles (4.8 km) to cool down.

148

LEVEL I
Close grip floor press 5-x-5
Dead hang from parallel bars 3 × :30
Front squat hold 3 × :20
Pushup 5-x-8

LEVEL II
Close grip floor press 7-x-1
Chinup from parallel bars 5-x-5
Front squat hold 3 × :20
Ring pushup 3-x-8

LEVEL III
Close grip floor press 10-x-1
Weighted chinup from parallel bars 8-x-3
Front squat hold 3 × :30
Ring pushup 5-x-8

NOTES: All weights are determined by the strength of the individual. The goal is to find the heaviest weight possible for the prescribed number of repetitions. However, do not sacrifice technique for load. If parallel bars are unavailable, use a standard pullup bar.

149

LEVEL I
Back squat 5-x-4
Rack pull deadlift 3-x-3
Situp 3-x-20
Good morning 3-x-10

LEVEL II
Back squat 7-x-2
Rack pull deadlift 4-x-3
Abmat situp 3-x-20
Single leg good morning 3-x-10

LEVEL III
Back squat 10-x-2
Rack pull deadlift 5-x-3
GHD situp 3-x-20
Single leg Romanian deadlift 3-x-10

NOTES: All weights are determined by the strength of the individual. The goal is to find the heaviest weight possible for the prescribed number of repetitions. However, do not sacrifice technique for load. Rack pull deadlifts should begin just below the knees with the bar supported on a rack or elevated surface. Romanian deadlift is a straight leg version of the deadlift.

150

LEVEL I
21-15-9 for time:
Pushup
Hang clean (95 pounds [43 kg]/65 pounds [29.5 kg])

LEVEL II
21-15-9 for time:
Hand release pushup
Hang clean (115 pounds [52 kg]/75 pounds [34 kg])

LEVEL III
21-15-9 for time:
Handstand pushup
Hang clean (135 pounds [61 kg]/95 pounds [43 kg])

NOTES: This is a sprint-style workout. Attempt to complete as much of the workout unbroken as possible. Handstand pushups may be kipped if necessary.

WODs AT THE GYM

151

LEVEL I
Hang snatch 5-x-3
Clean technique 10 minutes practice
Front squat 3-x-5

LEVEL II
Hang snatch 7-x-3
1 clean EMOTM 10 minutes at 80 percent 1RM
Front squat 4-x-5

LEVEL III
Hang snatch 10-x-3
1 clean every :30 at 90 percent 1RM for 10 minutes
Front squat 6-x-5

NOTES: All weights are determined by the strength of the individual. The goal is to find the heaviest weight possible for the prescribed number of repetitions. However, do not sacrifice technique for load. If an athlete doesn't know percentages, work to a heavy single clean and operate there for the duration of the workout.

152 (HOPE)

LEVEL I
1-minute each exercise for max repetitions:
Burpees
Power snatches (75 pounds [34 kg]/55 pounds [25 kg])
Box jumps
Thrusters (75 pounds [34 kg]/55 pounds [25 kg])
Jumping pullups

LEVEL II
1-minute each exercise for max repetitions:
Burpees
Power snatches (75 pounds [34 kg]/55 pounds [25 kg])
Box jumps
Thrusters (75 pounds [34 kg]/55 pounds [25 kg])
Chest to bar pullups
1-minute rest
Complete 2 rounds

LEVEL III
1-minute each exercise for max repetitions:
Burpees
Power snatches (75 pounds [34 kg]/55 pounds [25 kg])
Box jumps
Thrusters (75 pounds [34 kg]/55 pounds [25 kg])
Chest to bar pullups
1-minute rest
Complete 3 rounds

NOTES: This is a popular benchmark workout known as "Hope." The goal is to accumulate as many repetitions as possible over 3 rounds of the workout.

153

LEVEL I
Front squat 4-x-5
Sumo deadlift 4-x-5
Good morning 4-x-8
Bicycle crunch 3-x-20

LEVEL II
Front squat 7-x-1
Sumo deadlift 7-x-3
Barbell good morning 3-x-8
Lateral toes to bar 3-x-10

LEVEL III
Front squat 10-x-1
Sumo deadlift 10-x-3
Barbell good morning 4-x-8
Lateral toes to bar 4-x-10

NOTES: All weights are determined by the strength of the individual. The goal is to find the heaviest weight possible for the prescribed number of repetitions. However, do not sacrifice technique for load. Lateral toes to bar are like standard toes to bar except the toes contact the bar outside the grip on alternating sides.

154

LEVEL I
Push press 5-x-5
Ring row 3-x-10
Pushup 3-x-max
Hollow rock 3-x-20

LEVEL II
Push press 7-x-2
Seated row 4-x-10
Bar dip 4-x-max
Abmat situp 3-x-20

LEVEL III
Push press 10-x-2
Sled row 5-x-25-meters
Ring dip 5-x-max
GHD situp 3-x-20

NOTES: All weights are determined by the strength of the individual. The goal is to find the heaviest weight possible for the prescribed number of repetitions. However, do not sacrifice technique for load. Sled rows should be done facing the sled, rowing the weight toward the body, then backing up to repeat.

155

LEVEL I
30 miles (48 km) on stationary bike for time

LEVEL II
30 miles (48 km) on stationary bike for time

LEVEL III
30 miles (48 km) on stationary bike for time

NOTE: This is aerobic training, so the pace should be slow and steady.

WODs AT THE GYM

156

LEVEL I
Squat snatch 3-x-3
Power clean 10 minutes practice
Front squat 3-x-3

LEVEL II
1 squat snatch EMOTM 10 minutes at 80 percent 1RM
Power clean 7-x-1
Front squat 5-x-3

LEVEL III
1 squat snatch every :30 at 90 percent 1RM for 10 minutes
Power clean 10-x-1
Front squat 8-x-3

NOTES: If you don't know your percentages, work up to a heavy single, then perform snatches there. All other weights are determined by the strength of the individual. The goal is to find the heaviest weight possible for the prescribed number of repetitions. However, do not sacrifice technique for load.

157

LEVEL I
15-10-5 for time:
Overhead squat (45 pounds [20.5 kg]/35 pounds [16 kg])
Burpee over bar

LEVEL II
21-15-9 for time:
Overhead squat (75 pounds [34 kg]/55 pounds [25 kg])
Burpee over bar

LEVEL III
21-15-9 for time:
Overhead squat (95 pounds [43 kg]/65 pounds [29.5 kg])
Burpee over bar

NOTES: This is a sprint. Attempt to complete all sets unbroken. At level I, focus on form and depth during overhead squats especially.

158

LEVEL I
Box squat 4-x-5
Deficit deadlift 3-x-5
Sled pull 100-meters

LEVEL II
Box squat 3-x-3, 3-x-2, 3-x-1
Deficit deadlift 4-x-5
Sled pull 200-meters

LEVEL III
Box squat 3-x-3, 3-x-2, 3-x-1
Deficit deadlift 5-x-5
Sled pull 400-meters

NOTES: All weights are determined by the strength of the individual. The goal is to find the heaviest weight possible for the prescribed number of repetitions. However, do not sacrifice technique for load. Deficit deadlifts are performed by elevating the feet on a block while the weight remains on the ground. This increases the distance the bar is pulled during the lift.

159

LEVEL I
Floor press 5-x-5
Bent row 3-x-10
Step ups 3-x-10 each leg

LEVEL II
Floor press 7-x-2
Seated anchor drag 3-x-50 feet
Box jump 3-x-15

LEVEL III
Floor press 10-x-2
Seated anchor drag 3-x-50 feet
Box jump 3-x-20

NOTES: All weights are determined by the strength of the individual. The goal is to find the heaviest weight possible for the prescribed number of repetitions. However, do not sacrifice technique for load. Anchor drag is possible only if you a rope is available. If not, complete workout with bent rows.

160 (DT)

LEVEL I
3 rounds for time at 95 pounds (43 kg)/65 pounds (29.5 kg)
12 deadlifts
9 hang cleans
6 jerks

LEVEL II
4 rounds for time at 135 pounds (61 kg)/95 pounds (43 kg)
12 deadlifts
9 hang cleans
6 jerks

LEVEL III
5 rounds for time at 155 pounds (70.5 kg)/105 pounds (47.5 kg)
12 deadlifts
9 hang cleans
6 jerks

NOTES: This is a popular hero workout known as "DT." It is a medium weight lifting complex intended to be done quickly. Attempt to do each round unbroken if possible.

161

LEVEL I
Snatch 10 minutes practice
Hang clean 3-x-5

LEVEL II
Establish 1RM snatch
Hang clean 4-x-5

LEVEL III
Establish 1RM snatch
Hang clean 5-x-5

NOTES: This is a strength test. Use as many reps as necessary to establish the heaviest snatch you can perform successfully.

162

LEVEL I

EMOTM; 5-minutes:
3 rope climbs to standing
10 air squats

LEVEL II

EMOTM; 5-minutes:
1 rope climb
7 overhead squats (75 pounds [34 kg]/55 pounds [25 kg])

LEVEL III

EMOTM; 5-minutes:
1 rope climb
10 overhead squats (95 pounds [43 kg]/65 pounds [29.5 kg])

NOTES: This is a skill test. Complete each round quickly to allow enough time to rest before the next minute.

163

LEVEL I

EMOTM; 10-minutes:
5 ring rows
10 step ups

LEVEL II

EMOTM; 10-minutes:
5 pullups
10 box jumps

LEVEL III

EMOTM; 15-minutes:
5 chest to bar pullups
10 box jumps

NOTES: This is a skill test. Perform each set quickly to allow enough time to rest before the next minute. If a round is failed, rest the next minute, and then resume the workout.

164

LEVEL I

5-x-1 of press complex:
1 strict press + 2 push presses + 3 jerks
Bent row 3-x-6
Waiter's walk 1-x-100 each arm

LEVEL II

7-x-1 of press complex:
1 strict press + 2 push press + 3 jerk
Bent row 4-x-6
Waiter's walk 1-x-100 each arm

LEVEL III

10-x-1 of press complex:
1 strict press + 2 push press + 3 jerk
Bent row 5-x-6
Waiter's walk 2-x-100 each arm

NOTES: All weights are determined by the strength of the individual. The goal is to find the heaviest weight possible for the prescribed number of repetitions. However, do not sacrifice technique for load.

165

LEVEL I
Back squat 5-x-5
Deadlift 3-x-5
Good morning 3-x-8
Plank 2-x-max time

LEVEL II
5 back squat EMOTM 10 minutes at 70 percent 1RM
Deadlift 4-x-5
Good morning 3-x-10
Plank 3-x-max time

LEVEL III
5 back squat EMOTM 10 minutes at 70 percent 1RM
Deadlift with bands 5-x-5
Glute ham raise 3-x-8
Weighted plank 3-x-max time

NOTES: If athletes don't know percentages, work up to a medium weight for 5 back squats and complete the workout there. Deadlifts should be done with large rubber bands draped over the bar to provide additional tension. If no bands are available, complete workout without them.

166

LEVEL I
10-minute Airdyne for max distance

LEVEL II
10-minute Airdyne for max distance

LEVEL III
10-minute Airdyne for max distance

NOTES: This is an endurance test. The goal is to find a workable pace that is as near to maximum effort as possible without causing the body to fail.

167

LEVEL I
3-x-1 of the snatch complex:
3 snatch deadlift, 2 power snatch, 1 hang snatch

3-x-1 of the clean complex:
1 deadlift, 1 hang power clean, 1 squat clean, 1 jerk

LEVEL II
5-x-1 of the snatch complex:
3 snatch deadlift, 2 power snatch, 1 hang squat snatch

5-x-1 of the clean complex:
1 deadlift, 1 hang power clean, 1 squat clean, 1 jerk

LEVEL III
7-x-1 of the snatch complex:
3 snatch deadlift, 2 power snatch, 1 hang squat snatch

7-x-1 of the clean complex:
1 deadlift, 1 hang power clean, 1 squat clean, 1 jerk

NOTES: All weights are determined by the strength of the individual. The goal is to find the heaviest weight possible for the prescribed number of repetitions. However, do not sacrifice technique for load.

168 (FILTHY FIFTY)

LEVEL I

For time:
30 step ups
30 jumping pullups
30 kettlebell swings (35 pounds [16 kg])
30 walking lunges
30 push presses (45 pounds [20.5 kg])
30 situps
30 good mornings
30 ball slams
30 burpees
90 single unders

LEVEL II

For time:
40 box jumps
40 jumping pullups
40 kettlebell swings (35 pounds [16 kg])
40 walking lunges
40 push presses (45 pounds [20.5 kg])
40 knees to elbows
40 back extensions
40 wall balls
40 burpees
40 double unders

LEVEL III

For time:
50 box jumps
50 jumping pullups
50 kettlebell swings (35 pounds [16 kg])
50 walking lunges
50 push presses (45 pounds [20.5 kg])
50 knees to elbows
50 back extensions
50 wall balls
50 burpees
50 double unders

NOTES: This is a popular benchmark known as the "Filthy Fifty." The pace for this workout should be moderate and consistent. Medicine balls should weigh 20 pounds (9 kg) for men and 14 pounds (6.5 kg) for women, with a 10-foot (3 m) and 9-foot (2.7 m) target, respectively.

169

LEVEL I
5 rounds for completion:
5 kettlebell windmills each side
90 single unders

LEVEL II
5 rounds for completion:
5 kettlebell windmills each side
30 double unders

LEVEL III
5 rounds for completion:
5 kettlebell windmills each side
30 double unders

NOTES: This is a skill test with no time component. Focus should be on quality of reps rather than speed.

170

LEVEL I
Strict press 3-x-5
Push press 3-x-5
GHD situp 3-x-25
Thick bar curl 3-x-10

LEVEL II
3 strict presses EMOTM 5 minutes at 70 percent 1RM
3 push presses EMOTM 5 minutes at 1RM strict press
Abmat situp 3-x-25
Thick bar curl 3-x-10

LEVEL III
5 strict presses EMOTM 5 minutes at 70 percent 1RM
5 push presses EMOTM 5 minutes at 1RM strict press
GHD situp 3-x-25
Thick bar curl 3-x-10

NOTES: If you don't know your percentages, work up to a tough 5 rep strict press and complete the strict portion of the workout there. From that weight, add 30 percent and complete the push press portion of the workout.

171

LEVEL I
Back squat 5-x-3
Sumo deadlift rack pull 3-x-5
Weighted hip extension 3-x-10
Dumbbell row 3-x-10 each arm

LEVEL II
3 back squats EMOTM 10 minutes at 70 percent 1RM
Sumo deadlift rack pull 4-x-2
Weighted hip extension 3-x-10
Dumbbell row 3-x-10 each arm

LEVEL III
3 back squats EMOTM 15 minutes at 80 percent 1RM
Sumo deadlift rack pull 6-x-2
Weighted hip extension 3-x-10
Dumbbell row 3-x-10 each arm

NOTES: If you don't know your percentages, work up to a moderately heavy triple and complete the workout there. Rack pulls should be taken from just below the knee by placing the bar in a rack or on an elevation.

WODs AT THE GYM

172

LEVEL I
10 rounds for time:
5 jumping pullups
10 pushups
15 air squats

LEVEL II
10 rounds for time:
5 pullups
10 ring pushups
15 air squats

LEVEL III
10 rounds for time:
5 chest to bar pullups
10 ring pushups
15 pistol squats

NOTES: This is an endurance-style workout, so You will need to know what size sets they are capable of. The ultimate goal is to do all sets unbroken.

173

LEVEL I
15 minutes snatch practice
Front squat 1-x-20

LEVEL II
15-minutes to complete as much of the snatch ladder as possible:
10 snatches at 60 percent 1RM
10 snatches at 70 percent1RM
10 snatches at 80 percent 1RM
10 snatches at 90 percent 1RM
Front squat 1-x-20

LEVEL III
15-minutes to complete as much of the snatch ladder as possible:
10 snatches at 60 percent 1RM
10 snatches at 70 percent1RM
10 snatches at 80 percent 1RM
10 snatches at 90 percent 1RM
Front squat 1-x-20

NOTES: If you don't know your percentages, use 10 minutes to establish a 1RM snatch and base all weights off of that.

174

LEVEL I
EMOTM; 10-minutes:
1 deadlift
1 hang clean
1 squat clean
1 jerk

LEVEL II
EMOTM; 10-minutes:
1 deadlift
1 hang clean
1 squat clean
1 jerk

LEVEL III
EMOTM; 10-minutes:
1 deadlift
1 hang clean
1 squat clean
1 jerk

NOTES: All weights are determined by the strength of the individual. The goal is to find the heaviest weight possible for the prescribed number of repetitions. However, do not sacrifice technique for load. All movements should be completed without dropping the bar.

175

LEVEL I
For time:
50 floor presses at ½ bodyweight
25 push presses at ½ bodyweight
25 push jerks at ½ bodyweight

LEVEL II
For time:
50 floor presses at ¾ bodyweight
25 push presses at ¾ bodyweight
25 push jerks at ¾ bodyweight

LEVEL III
For time:
50 floor presses at bodyweight
25 push presses at bodyweight
25 push jerks at bodyweight

NOTES: If you are unable to complete the workout as written due to strength/bodyweight ratio, scale down the weight until doable.

176

LEVEL I
Back squat 5-x-5
Deadlift 3-x-5
Back extension 3-x-10
Ring row 3-x-10

LEVEL II
1 back squat EMOTM 20 minutes at 80 percent 1RM
Deadlift 5-x-2 for speed
Back extension 3-x-10
Bent row 3-x-10

LEVEL III
1 back squat EMOTM 20 minutes at 90 percent 1RM
Deadlift 7-x-2 for speed
Glute ham raise 4-x-10
Bent row 4-x-10

NOTES: If you don't know your percentages, work to a heavy single and complete workout there. All other weights are determined by the strength of the individual. The goal is to find the heaviest weight possible for the prescribed number of repetitions. However, do not sacrifice technique for load.

177

LEVEL I
Clean 5-x-3
Front squat 3-x-6

LEVEL II
For time:
10 cleans at 60 percent 1RM
10 cleans at 70 percent 1RM
10 cleans at 80 percent 1RM
10 cleans at 90 percent 1RM
Front squats 3-x-6

LEVEL III
For time:
10 cleans at 60 percent 1RM
10 cleans at 70 percent 1RM
10 cleans at 80 percent 1RM
10 cleans at 90 percent 1RM
Front squat 4-x-6

NOTES: If you don't know your percentages, use 10 minutes to establish a 1RM clean and base all weights off of that.

WODs AT THE GYM

178

LEVEL I
For time:
Row 2000-meters
50 jumping pullups
50 pushups
50 step ups
Row 2000-meters

LEVEL II
For time:
Row 2000-meters
50 pullups
50 bar dips
50 box jumps
Row 2000-meters

LEVEL III
For time:
Row 2000-meters
75 pullups
75 ring dips
75 box jumps
Row 2000-meters

NOTES: This is a high-volume workout, so don't go out too fast. The bodyweight movements are going to need to be broken into smaller sets, based on ability level. The goal is to keep rest periods short.

179

LEVEL I
Complete 5 rounds of the snatch complex:
1 snatch deadlift
1 hang power snatch
1 squat snatch

LEVEL II
Complete 7 rounds of the snatch complex:
1 snatch deadlift
1 hang power snatch
1 squat snatch

LEVEL III
Complete 10 rounds of the snatch complex:
1 snatch deadlift
1 hang power snatch
1 squat snatch

NOTES: All weights are determined by the strength of the individual. The goal is to find the heaviest weight possible for the prescribed number of repetitions. However, do not sacrifice technique for load. Do not drop the bar between exercises.

180

LEVEL I
EMOTM; 10-minutes:
5 jumping pullups
10 hollow rocks

LEVEL II
EMOTM; 10-minutes:
1 bar muscle ups
15 hollow rocks

LEVEL III
EMOTM; 10-minutes:
3 bar muscle ups
20 hollow rocks

NOTES: This is a skill test. You will need to finish each round quickly to allow for enough time to rest before the next minute.

181

LEVEL I
Complete 5 rounds of the clean complex:
1 deadlift
1 hang power clean
1 squat clean
1 jerk

LEVEL II
Complete 7 rounds of the clean complex:
1 deadlift
1 hang power clean
1 squat clean
1 jerk

LEVEL III
Complete 10 rounds of the clean complex:
1 deadlift
1 hang power clean
1 squat clean
1 jerk

NOTES: All weights are determined by the strength of the individual. The goal is to find the heaviest weight possible for the prescribed number of repetitions. However, do not sacrifice technique for load. Do not drop the bar between exercises.

182

LEVEL I
10-minute AMRAP:
5 floor presses at ½ bodyweight
15 pushups

LEVEL II
10-minute AMRAP:
5 floor presses at bodyweight
15 pushups

LEVEL III
10-minute AMRAP:
5 floor presses at 1¼ bodyweight
15 pushups

NOTES: If you are unable to complete the workout due to strength/bodyweight ratio, scale weight down until it is doable.

183

LEVEL I
10-minute AMRAP:
5 push presses at ½ bodyweight
10 hand release pushups

LEVEL II
10-minute AMRAP:
5 push presses at ¾ bodyweight
10 piked pushups

LEVEL III
10-minute AMRAP:
5 push presses at bodyweight
10 handstand pushups

NOTES: If you are unable to complete the workout due to strength/bodyweight ratio, scale weight down until it is doable.

WODs AT THE GYM

184

LEVEL I
10-minute AMRAP:
5 jerks at ½ bodyweight
5 jumping pullups

LEVEL II
10-minute AMRAP:
5 jerks at ¾ bodyweight
5 chest to bar pullups

LEVEL III
10-minute AMRAP:
5 jerks at 1¼ bodyweight
5 muscle ups

NOTES: If you are unable to complete workout due to strength/bodyweight ratio, scale weight down until it is doable.

185

LEVEL I
Back squat 3-x-5
Conventional deadlift 3-x-3
Barbell good morning 3-x-12
Bent row 3-x-12

LEVEL II
Back squat with chains 4-x-5
Sumo deadlift 4-x-3
Barbell good morning 3-x-12
Bent row 3-x-12

LEVEL III
Box squat with chains 5-x-5
Stone deadlift 5-x-3
Barbell good morning 3-x-12
Bent row 3-x-12

NOTES: All weights are determined by the strength of the individual. The goal is to find the heaviest weight possible for the prescribed number of repetitions. However, do not sacrifice technique for load. If chains are unavailable, complete workout without. Any stone will work for the deadlifts.

186

LEVEL I
2 rounds for time:
400-meter run
21 wall balls
15 jumping pullups
9 pushups

LEVEL II
3 rounds for time:
400-meter run
21 wall balls
15 pullups
9 piked pushups

LEVEL III
3 rounds for time:
400-meter run
21 wall balls
15 chest to bar pullups
9 handstand pushups from deficit

NOTES: Medicine balls should be 20 pounds (9 kg) for men and 14 pounds (6.5 kg) for women, with 10-foot (3 m) and 9-foot (2.7 m) targets, respectively. Handstand pushup deficit can be created using parallettes or blocks.

187

LEVEL I

10 rounds for completion (55 pounds [25 kg]/35 pounds [16 kg]):
1 power snatch
1 snatch balance
1 oh squat
1 full snatch

LEVEL II

10 rounds for time (95 pounds [43 kg]/65 pounds [29.5 kg]):
1 power snatch
1 snatch balance
1 oh squat
1 full snatch

LEVEL III

10 rounds for time (115 pounds [52 kg]/75 pounds [34 kg]):
1 power snatch
1 snatch balance
1 oh squat
1 full snatch

NOTES: At level I, focus on quality over speed. At level II and level III, focus on efficiency and speed.

188 (Diane)

LEVEL I

21-15-9 for time:
Deadlifts (135 pounds [61 kg]/95 pounds [43 kg])
Hand release pushups

LEVEL II

21-15-9 for time:
Deadlifts (185 pounds [84 kg]/125 pounds [56.5 kg])
Piked pushups

LEVEL III

21-15-9 for time:
Deadlifts (225 pounds [102 kg]/155 pounds [70.5 kg])
Handstand pushups

NOTES: This is a popular benchmark workout known as "Diane." It is a sprint-style workout for those who can do handstand pushups easily. For those who struggle, it is more paced and calculated. Kipping is allowed.

189

LEVEL I

Back squat 3-x-5
Deadlift 5-x-2
Good morning 3-x-10
Farmer's Carry-3-x-50-meters slow walk

LEVEL II

Back squat 4-x-5 with :03 pause at bottom
Deadlift 7-x-2
Barbell good morning 3-x-10
Farmer's Carry-3-x-50-meters slow walk

LEVEL III

Back squat 5-x-5 with :03 pause at bottom
Deadlift 10-x-2
Barbell good morning 3-x-10
Farmer's Carry-3-x-50-meters slow walk

NOTES: All weights are determined by the strength of the individual. The goal is to find the heaviest weight possible for the prescribed number of repetitions. However, do not sacrifice technique for load.

190

LEVEL I

Every 2 minutes for 10 minutes complete:
3 strict presses
6 push presses
Situp 4-×-10
Overhead hold for max time (45 pounds [20.5 kg]/35 pounds [16 kg])

LEVEL II

Every 2 minutes for 14 minutes complete:
3 strict press
6 push press
GHD situp 3-×-15
Overhead hold for max time (95 pounds [43 kg]/65 pounds [29.5 kg])

LEVEL III

Every 2 minutes for 20 minutes complete:
3 strict press
6 push press
GHD situp 4-×-20
Overhead hold for max time (115 pounds [52 kg]/75 pounds [34 kg])

NOTES: All weights are determined by the strength of the individual. The goal is to find the heaviest weight possible for the prescribed number of repetitions. However, do not sacrifice technique for load.

191

LEVEL I

3-minute AMRAP single unders
3-minute AMRAP power snatches

LEVEL II

4-minute AMRAP double unders
4-minute AMRAP squat snatches (95 pounds [43 kg]/65 pounds [29.5 kg])

LEVEL III

5-minute AMRAP double unders
5-minute AMRAP squat snatches (95 pounds [43 kg]/65 pounds [29.5 kg])

NOTES: Do not rest between exercises. The goal of this workout is to maintain good technique while tired. Score is total reps completed.

192

LEVEL I

Establish 1RM snatch
Establish 1RM clean and jerk

LEVEL II

Establish 1RM snatch
Establish 1RM clean and jerk

LEVEL III

Establish 1RM snatch
Establish 1RM clean and jerk

NOTES: This is a strength test. Use as many attempts as they feel necessary to establish their 1RMs.

193 (Isabel/Grace)

LEVEL I

For completion:
30 snatches (55 pounds
[25 kg]/35 pounds [16 kg])
30 clean and jerks (55 pounds
[25 kg]/35 pounds [16 kg])

LEVEL II

For time:
30 snatches (95 pounds
[43 kg]/65 pounds [29.5 kg])
30 clean and jerks (95 pounds
[43 kg]/65 pounds [29.5 kg])

LEVEL III

For time:
30 snatches (135 pounds
[61 kg]/95 pounds [43 kg])
30 clean and jerks (135 pounds
[61 kg]/95 pounds [43 kg])

NOTES: This is a combination of
two popular benchmarks known as
"Isabel" and "Grace." At level I,
attempt to perform all movements
perfectly. At level II and level III,
focus on efficiency and strategy for
how often to break up the sets.

194

LEVEL I

For time:
30 ring rows
30 jumping pullups
30 pushups

LEVEL II

For time:
30 ring dips
30 chest to bar pullups
30 piked pushups

LEVEL III

For time:
30 ring muscle ups
30 bar muscle ups
30 handstand pushups

NOTES: This is a high-volume
muscular endurance workout. You will
need to know when to break up the
sets and how long to rest.

195

LEVEL I

Accumulate 3 minutes in the
bottom of an overhead squat
Accumulate 3 minutes in the
bottom of a front squat

LEVEL II

Accumulate 4 minutes in the
bottom of an overhead squat
Accumulate 4 minutes in the
bottom of a front squat

LEVEL III

Accumulate 5 minutes in the
bottom of an overhead squat
Accumulate 5 minutes in the
bottom of a front squat

NOTES: All weights are determined
by the strength of the individual.
Weights do not need to be heavy
here, since the goal is positioning
and flexibility. This is a great way to
improve comfort at the bottom of a
squat. Time may be accumulated in
as many intervals as needed.

WODs AT THE GYM

196

LEVEL I
EMOTM 20 minutes for form:
Odd minutes: 5 deadlifts
Even minutes: 5 hang cleans

LEVEL II
EMOTM; 14 minutes:
Odd minutes: 5 deadlifts at 70 percent 1RM
Even minutes: 5 hang cleans at 70 percent 1RM

LEVEL III
EMOTM; 20-minutes:
Odd minutes: 5 deadlifts at 70 percent 1RM
Even minutes: 5 hang cleans at 70 percent 1RM

NOTES: If you don't know your percentages, work up to a moderately heavy 5 reps for deadlift and complete the deadlift portion there. Do the same for hang cleans.

197

LEVEL I
Bench press 3-x-5 with pause
Romanian deadlift + bent row 3-x-6
200-meter overhead carry (45 pounds [20.5 kg]/35 pounds [16 kg])

LEVEL II
Bench press 4-x-5 with pause
Romanian deadlift + bent row 4-x-6
400-meter overhead carry (95 pounds [43 kg]/65 pounds [29.5 kg])

LEVEL III
Bench press 5-x-5 with pause
Romanian deadlift + bent row 6-x-6
400-meter overhead carry 115 pounds [52 kg]/75 pounds [34 kg])

NOTES: All weights are determined by the strength of the individual. The goal is to find the heaviest weight possible for the prescribed number of repetitions. However, do not sacrifice technique for load.

198

LEVEL I
For completion:
15 snatches at 60 percent 1RM
12 snatches at 70 percent 1RM
9 snatch at 80 percent 1RM
6 snatch at 90 percent 1RM
3 snatch at 100 percent 1RM

LEVEL II
For time with 20-minute cap:
15 snatches at 60 percent 1RM
12 snatches at 70 percent 1RM
9 snatches at 80 percent 1RM
6 snatches at 90 percent 1RM
3 snatch at 100 percent 1RM

LEVEL III
For time with 15-minute cap:
15 snatches at 60 percent 1RM
12 snatches at 70 percent 1RM
9 snatches at 80 percent 1RM
6 snatches at 90 percent 1RM
3 snatches at 100 percent 1RM

NOTES: If you don't know your percentages, use 10 minutes to establish a 1RM snatch and base all weights off that number.

199

LEVEL I
20 perfect hang clean and jerks
Front squat 3-x-10

LEVEL II
25 perfect hang clean and jerks
Front squat 4-x-10

LEVEL III
30 perfect hang clean and jerks
Front squat 5-x-10

NOTES: Use any weight for clean and jerks because they are strictly for form. Front squats should be built up to the heaviest possible for 10 reps.

200

LEVEL I
For completion:
15 cleans at 60 percent 1RM
12 cleans at 70 percent 1RM
9 cleans at 80 percent 1RM
6 cleans at 90 percent 1RM
3 cleans at 100 percent 1RM

LEVEL II
For time with 20-minute cap:
15 cleans at 60 percent 1RM
12 cleans at 70 percent 1RM
9 cleans at 80 percent 1RM
6 cleans at 90 percent 1RM
3 cleans at 100 percent 1RM

LEVEL III
For time with 15-minute cap:
15 cleans at 60 percent 1RM
12 cleans at 70 percent 1RM
9 cleans at 80 percent 1RM
6 cleans at 90 percent 1RM
3 cleans at 100 percent 1RM

NOTES: If you don't know your percentages, use 10 minutes to establish 1RM clean and base all weights off that number.

WODs AT THE GYM

201

LEVEL I
20 perfect snatches
Overhead squat 3-x-10

LEVEL II
30 perfect snatches
Overhead squat 4-x-10

LEVEL III
30 perfect snatches
Overhead squat 5-x-10

NOTES: Use any weight for snatches. Only form matters. Overhead squats should be loaded increasingly until heaviest weight for 10 reps is reached.

202

LEVEL I
Compete 5 rounds of the complex:
1 strict press
3 push presses
5 split jerk
Pushups 5-x-max
Situps 3-x-20
200-meter waiter's walk each arm

LEVEL II
Compete 7 rounds of the complex:
1 strict press
3 push presses
5 split jerk
Bar dips 5-x-max
Abmat situps 3-x-20
300-meter waiter's walk each arm

LEVEL III
Compete 10 rounds of the complex:
1 strict press
3 push presses
5 split jerk
Ring dips 5-x-max
GHD situps 3-x-20
400-meter waiter's walk each arm

NOTES: All weights are determined by the strength of the individual. The goal is to find the heaviest weight possible for the prescribed number of repetitions. However, do not sacrifice technique for load.

203

LEVEL I
3 minutes max single unders
Accumulate 3 minutes in bottom of front squat
3 minutes max box jump

LEVEL II
4 minutes max double unders
Accumulate 4 minutes in bottom of front squat
4 minutes max box jump

LEVEL III
5 minutes max double unders
Accumulate 5 minutes in bottom of front squat
5 minutes max box jump

NOTE: The weight for front squat hold does not need to be heavy.

204

LEVEL I
10 rounds for time:
1 deadlift (185 pounds [84 kg]/125 pounds [56.5 kg])
5 pushups

LEVEL II
10 rounds for time:
1 deadlift (225 pounds [102 kg]/155 pounds [70.5 kg])
5 piked pushups

LEVEL III
10 rounds for time:
1 deadlift (315 pounds [143 kg]/225 pounds [102 kg])
5 handstand pushups

NOTES: This is meant to be a fast and heavy conditioning workout. Attempt to complete it unbroken.

205

LEVEL I
Floor press 3-x-6
Strict chinup 3-x-6
Pushups 2-x-max
Toes to bar 3-x-10

LEVEL II
Floor press 4-x-6
Strict chinup 4-x-6
Pushups 3-x-max
Toes to bar 3-x-15

LEVEL III
Floor press 5-x-6
Strict chinup 5-x-6
Pushups 4-x-max
Toes to bar 4-x-20

NOTES: All weights are determined by the strength of the individual. The goal is to find the heaviest weight possible for the prescribed number of repetitions. However, do not sacrifice technique for load.

WODs AT THE GYM

206 (AMANDA)

LEVEL I
15-10-5 for time:
Jumping pullup
Power snatch (75 pounds
[34 kg]/55 pounds [25 kg])

LEVEL II
9-7-5 for time:
Muscle up
Squat snatch (95 pounds
[43 kg]/65 pounds [29.5 kg])

LEVEL III
9-7-5 for time:
Muscle up
Squat snatch (135 pounds
[61 kg]/95 pounds [43 kg])

NOTES: This is a popular
benchmark known as "Amanda." With
good muscle ups, attempt to do them
unbroken. If you struggle with muscle
ups should break them into smaller
sets. The same goes for the snatches.

207

LEVEL I
5 rounds for completion:
:30 squat hold
:15 V sit hold
5 wall walks

LEVEL II
7 rounds for completion:
:30 oh squat hold
:15 L sit hold
5 kicks to wall handstand

LEVEL III
10 rounds for completion:
:30 oh squat hold
:15 L sit hold
5 kicks to handstand

NOTES: This is a skill test with no
time component. The weight of the
squat hold is not important. L sits may
be done hanging or from support.

208

LEVEL I
For time:
40 back squats (95 pounds
[43 kg]/65 pounds [29.5 kg])
20 shoulder to overheads
30 jumping pullups

LEVEL II
For time:
40 back squats (135 pounds
[61 kg]/95 pounds [43 kg])
20 shoulder to overheads
30 pullups

LEVEL III
For time:
50 back squats (135 pounds
[61 kg]/95 pounds [43 kg])
30 shoulder to overheads
40 pullups

NOTES: This is a high-volume
workout. Pace the squats and
shoulder to overheads so as not to
burn the arms out for the pullups.

209

LEVEL I

Establish 1RM bench press
Complete 30 reps at 60 percent 1RM (3-minute time cap)
Battling ropes 3-x-1:00
Situp 3-x-10

LEVEL II

Establish 1RM bench press
Complete 40 reps at 60 percent 1RM (3-minute time cap)
Battling ropes 3-x-1:00
Abmat situp 3-x-20

LEVEL III

Establish 1RM bench press
Complete 60 reps at 60 percent 1RM (3-minute time cap)
Battling ropes 3-x-1:00
GHD situp 3-x-20

NOTE: If ropes are unavailable, substitute ball slams.

210 (NANCY)

LEVEL I

3 rounds for time:
400-meter run
15 overhead squats (45 pounds [20.5 kg]/35 pounds [16 kg])

LEVEL II

4 rounds for time:
400-meter run
15 overhead squats (75 pounds [34 kg]/55 pounds [25 kg])

LEVEL III

5 rounds for time:
400-meter run
15 overhead squats (95 pounds [43 kg]/65 pounds [29.5 kg])

NOTES: This is a popular benchmark known as "Nancy." At level I, take their time on the overhead squats and focus on form and depth. At level II and level III, attempt to do all sets unbroken.

211

LEVEL I

3 rounds for time:
7 hang cleans (95 pounds [43 kg]/65 pounds [29.5 kg])
14 air squats

LEVEL II

3 rounds for time:
7 hang cleans (135 pounds [61 kg]/95 pounds [43 kg])
14 assisted pistol squats

LEVEL III

3 rounds for time:
7 hang cleans (225 pounds [102 kg]/135 pounds [61 kg])
14 pistol squats

NOTES: This is meant to be a heavy conditioning workout. The most difficult part may be holding on to the bar, so you will need to be strategic about how many consecutive reps you attempt.

WODs AT THE GYM

212

LEVEL I
10-minute AMRAP:
5 squat cleans (95 pounds [43 kg]/65 pounds [29.5 kg])
15 step ups

LEVEL II
10-minute AMRAP:
5 squat cleans (135 pounds [61 kg]/95 pounds [43 kg])
15 box jumps

LEVEL III
15-minute AMRAP:
5 squat cleans (185 pounds [84 kg]/115 pounds [52 kg])
15 box jumps

NOTES: This is a moderate-paced workout, so do not go out too fast. The goal is to keep a consistent pace with minimal rest.

213

LEVEL I
3 rounds for time:
4 rope climbs to standing
4 front squats (95 pounds [43 kg]/65 pounds [29.5 kg])

LEVEL II
3 rounds for time:
2 rope climbs
4 squat cleans (155 pounds [70.5 kg]/105 pounds [47.5 kg])

LEVEL III
3 rounds for time:
2 rope climbs
4 squat cleans (225 pounds [102 kg]/135 pounds 61 kg])

NOTES: This is a sprint. If ropes are unavailable, substitute 7 pullups per rope climb.

214

LEVEL I
12-minute AMRAP:
1-mile (1.6 km) Airdyne
50 box step overs
30 jumping pullups

LEVEL II
12-minute AMRAP:
1-mile (1.6 km) Airdyne
50 box jump overs
30 chest to bar pullups

LEVEL III
12-minute AMRAP:
1-mile (1.6 km) Airdyne
50 box jump overs
30 bar muscle ups

NOTES: This really is a for-time workout, but if you finish too quickly, hop back on the Airdyne. The pace should be moderate and steady; 12 minutes is a long time for these movements.

215

LEVEL I
Snatch 10 minutes practice
Complete 20 back squats
Complete 20 overhead squats

LEVEL II
Establish 1RM snatch
Complete 15 back squats at 1RM snatch
Complete 15 overhead squats at 75 percent 1RM snatch

LEVEL III
Establish 1RM snatch
Complete 20 back squats at 1RM snatch
Complete 20 overhead squats at 75 percent 1RM snatch

NOTES: At level II and level III, use no more than 20 minutes to establish 1RM snatch.

216

LEVEL I
50 burpees + 500 single unders for time
EMOTM during burpees complete 1 power snatch (55 pounds [25 kg]/35 pounds [16 kg])
EMOTM during double unders complete 1 overhead squats (55 pounds [25 kg]/35 pounds [16 kg])

LEVEL II
75 burpees + 250 double unders for time
EMOTM during burpees complete 5 power snatches (75 pounds [34 kg]/55 pounds [25 kg])
EMOTM during double unders complete 5 overhead squats (75 pounds [34 kg]/55 pounds [25 kg])

LEVEL III
100 burpees + 500 double unders for time
EMOTM during burpees complete 5 power snatches (95 pounds [43 kg]/65 pounds [29.5 kg])
EMOTM during double unders complete 5 overhead squats (95 pounds [43 kg]/65 pounds [29.5 kg])

NOTES: This is a major conditioning test. Every minute, you are required to perform the barbell work before accumulating the burpees or double unders. Time cap for this workout is 40 minutes.

217

LEVEL I
2 rounds for completion:
5 front squats
5 overhand deadlifts
20-meter lateral front rack carry
10 good mornings

LEVEL II
3 rounds for completion:
5 front squats at 80 percent 1RM
5 deadlifts at 1RM clean
20-meter lateral front rack carry
10 back extensions

LEVEL III
4 rounds for completion:
5 front squats at 80 percent 1RM
5 overhand deadlifts at 1RM clean
20-meter lateral front rack carry
10 weighted back extensions

NOTES: If you don't know your percentages work to a heavy 5 and complete front squats. Do the same for deadlifts. The lateral front rack carry should be 10-meters sliding right and 10-meters sliding left.

WODs AT THE GYM

218

LEVEL I
10-minute AMRAP:
1000-meter row
50 jumping pullups
50-meter front rack lunge
(45 pounds [20.5 kg]/35 pounds
[16 kg])

LEVEL II
12-minute AMRAP:
1000-meter row
50 pullups
50-meter front rack lunge
(95 pounds [43 kg]/65 pounds
[29.5 kg])

LEVEL III
15-minute AMRAP:
1000-meter row
50 chest to bar pullups
50-meter front rack lunge (135
pounds [61 kg]/95 pounds [43 kg])

NOTES: This is a high-volume
workout, so don't go out too fast
on the rower. You will need to know
how to break up the pullups so as to
minimize rest times.

219

LEVEL I
3 rounds for time:
5 deadlifts (135 pounds [61 kg]/95
pounds [43 kg])
20 burpees over bar

LEVEL II
4 rounds for time:
5 deadlifts (225 pounds [102
kg]/135 pounds [61 kg])
20 burpees over bar

LEVEL III
5 rounds for time:
5 deadlifts (315 pounds [143
kg]/225 pounds [102 kg])
20 burpees over bar

NOTES: This is a moderate-paced
workout. Attempt to do all sets
unbroken. The key is to maintain a
steady pace on the burpees.

220

LEVEL I
21-15-9 for time:
Wall balls
Jumping pullups
Pushups

LEVEL II
21-15-9 for time:
Wall balls
Pullups
Pushups

LEVEL III
21-15-9 for time:
Wall balls
Chest to bar pullups
Pushups

NOTES: This is a sprint. At level II
and level III, do all sets unbroken.

221

LEVEL I
20-minute AMRAP:
50 jumping pullups
800-meter run
50 dumbbell swings (45 pounds [20.5 kg]/25 pounds [11.5 kg])

LEVEL II
20-minute AMRAP:
50 pullups
800-meter run
50 alternating dumbbell snatches (55 pounds [25 kg]/35 pounds [16 kg])

LEVEL III
20-minute AMRAP:
100 pullups
800-meter run
100 alternating dumbbell snatches (75 pounds [34 kg]/55 pounds [25 kg])

NOTES: This is a high-volume workout, so you will need to know how to break up the sets to minimize muscle fatigue and rest times. At level I, do Russian-style swings (eye level).

222

LEVEL I
Clean and jerk 20 minutes practice
For completion:
15 back squats
15 front squats

LEVEL II
E2MOTM for 20-minutes:
1 clean and jerk
In less than 6 minutes complete:
15 back squats at 1RM clean and jerk
15 front squats at 75 percent 1RM clean and jerk

LEVEL III
E2MOTM for 20-minutes:
1 clean and jerk
In less than 4 minutes complete:
15 back squats at 1RM clean and jerk
15 front squats at 75 percent 1RM clean and jerk

NOTES: All weights are determined by the strength of the individual. The goal is to find the heaviest weight possible for the prescribed number of repetitions. However, do not sacrifice technique for load.

223

LEVEL I
Perform an increasing number of jumping pullups each minute:
1 jumping pullup in minute 1
2 jumping pullups in minute 2
3 jumping pullups in minute 3
(and so forth)

LEVEL II
Perform an increasing number of pullups each minute:
1 pullup in minute 1
2 pullups in minute 2
3 pullups in minute 3
(and so forth)

LEVEL III
Perform an increasing number of chest to bar pullups each minute:
1 chest to bar pullup in minute 1
2 chest to bar pullups in minute 2
3 chest to bar pullups in minute 3
(and so forth)

NOTES: Perform sets quickly to give yourself enough time to rest for the next minute.

WODs AT THE GYM

224

LEVEL I
8-minute AMRAP:
10 burpees
15 kettlebell swings
20 wall balls

LEVEL II
10-minute AMRAP:
10 burpees
15 kettlebell swings
20 wall balls

LEVEL III
12-minute AMRAP:
10 burpees
15 kettlebell swings
20 wall balls

NOTES: At level I, do Russian-style swings (eye level); At level II and level III, do American-style swings (overhead). Medicine balls should be 20 pounds (9 kg) for men and 14 pounds (6.5 kg) for women, with 10-foot (3 m) and 9-foot (2.7 m) targets, respectively.

225

LEVEL I
Snatch 3-x-1 at 95 percent 1RM
1 clean and jerk E2MOTM for 10 minutes at 80 percent 1RM

LEVEL II
Snatch 4-x-1 at 95 percent 1RM
1 clean and jerk E2MOTM for 15 minutes at 80 percent 1RM

LEVEL III
Snatch 5-x-1 at 95 percent 1RM
1 clean and jerk E2MOTM for 20 minutes at 80 percent 1RM

NOTES: If you don't know your percentages, work up to a heavy single snatch and complete the workout there. Do the same for clean and jerks.

226

LEVEL I
Clean and jerk 3-x-1 at 95 percent 1RM
1 snatch EMOTM for 6 minutes at 80 percent 1RM

LEVEL II
Clean and jerk 4-x-1 at 95 percent 1RM
1 snatch EMOTM for 8 minutes at 80 percent 1RM

LEVEL III
Clean and jerk 5-x-1 at 95 percent 1RM
1 snatch EMOTM for 10 minutes at 80 percent 1RM

NOTES: If you don't know your percentages, work up to a heavy clean and jerk and complete the workout there. Do the same for snatches.

227

LEVEL I
5 rounds for completion:
10 ring rows
10 jumping pullups
10 air squats

LEVEL II
7 rounds for completion:
5 strict pullups
5 kipping pullups
5 butterfly pullups
15 air squats

LEVEL III
10 rounds for completion:
5 strict pullups
5 kipping pullups
5 butterfly pullups
15 air squats

NOTES: This is a skill test with no time component. Focus on technique and fluidity.

228

LEVEL I
10-minute AMRAP:
200-meter run
10 push presses (75 pounds [34 kg]/55 pounds [25 kg])
15 step ups

LEVEL II
12-minute AMRAP:
200-meter run
10 push presses (95 pounds [43 kg]/65 pounds [29.5 kg])
15 box jumps

LEVEL III
15-minute AMRAP:
200-meter run
10 push presses (115 pounds [52 kg]/75 pounds [34 kg])
15 box jumps

NOTES: This is a moderate-paced workout, so no need to go out fast. At level II and level III, attempt to complete all sets unbroken.

229

LEVEL I
20-minute AMRAP:
2-mile (3.2 km) Airdyne
800-meter row
400-meter run
50 wall balls

LEVEL II
20-minute AMRAP:
2-mile (3.2 km) Airdyne
1200-meter row
600-meter run
75 wall balls

LEVEL III
20-minute AMRAP:
2-mile (3.2 km) Airdyne
1600-meter row
800-meter run
100 wall balls

NOTES: This is an endurance test with wall balls at the end of it. You will need to move quickly between exercises and stay consistent in order to finish. Men use a 20-pound (9 kg) ball to a 10-foot (3 m) target; women use a 14-pound (6.5 kg) ball to a 9-foot (2.7 m) target.

WODs AT THE GYM

230

LEVEL I
AMRAP; no breaks between

5-minute AMRAP:

5 thrusters (65 pounds [29.5 kg]/45 pounds [20.5 kg])

5 sumo deadlift high pulls (65 pounds [29.5 kg]/45 pounds [20.5 kg])

5 jumping pullups

3 minute AMRAP:

3 thrusters (65 pounds [29.5 kg]/45 pounds [20.5 kg])

3 sumo deadlift high pulls (65 pounds [29.5 kg]/45 pounds [20.5 kg])

3 jumping pullups

1-minute AMRAP:

1 thruster (65 pounds [29.5 kg]/45 pounds [20.5 kg])

1 sumo deadlift high pull (65 pounds [29.5 kg]/45 pounds [20.5 kg])

1 jumping pullup

LEVEL II
AMRAP; no breaks between

5-minute AMRAP:

5 thrusters (75 pounds [34 kg]/55 pounds [25 kg])

5 sumo deadlift high pulls (75 pounds [34 kg]/55 pounds [25 kg])

5 pullups

3 minute AMRAP:

3 thrusters (75 pounds [34 kg]/55 pounds [25 kg])

3 sumo deadlift high pulls (75 pounds [34 kg]/55 pounds [25 kg])

3 pullups

1-minute AMRAP:

1 thruster (75 pounds [34 kg]/55 pounds [25 kg])

1 sumo deadlift high pull (75 pounds [34 kg]/55 pounds [25 kg])

1 pullup

LEVEL III
AMRAP; no breaks between

5-minute AMRAP:

5 thrusters (95 pounds [43 kg]/65 pounds [29.5 kg])

5 sumo deadlift high pulls (95 pounds [43 kg]/65 pounds [29.5 kg])

5 chest to bar pullups

3 minute AMRAP:

3 thrusters (95 pounds [43 kg]/65 pounds [29.5 kg])

3 sumo deadlift high pulls (95 pounds [43 kg]/65 pounds [29.5 kg])

3 chest to bar pullups

1-minute AMRAP:

1 thruster (95 pounds [43 kg]/65 pounds [29.5 kg])

1 sumo deadlift high pull (95 pounds [43 kg]/65 pounds [29.5 kg])

1 chest to bar pullup

NOTES: This workout will last 9 minutes, but is broken into three sections. The 5-minute section requires sets of 5, the 3-minute section requires sets of 3, and the 1-minute section requires sets of 1. The score is total number of reps completed.

231

LEVEL I
For time:
75 wall balls
50 abmat situps
30 pushups
10 ring rows
10 assisted ring dips

LEVEL II
For time:
100 wall balls
50 knees to elbows
30 piked pushups
10 chest to bar pullups

LEVEL III
For time:
150 wall balls
50 toes to bar
30 handstand pushups
10 muscle ups

NOTES: This is a high-volume workout, so break up your sets according to your ability. At level I, use a band to assist with ring dips. Handstand pushups may be kipped, if necessary.

232

LEVEL I
Deadlift 3-x-5
Cleans 10 minutes practice
Walking lunge 3-x-20-meters

LEVEL II
Deadlift 4-x-5
Establish 10RM power clean
Front rack lunge 3-x-20-meters

LEVEL III
Deadlift 5-x-5
Establish 10RM power clean
Front rack lunge 4-x-20-meters

NOTES: All weights are determined by the strength of the individual. The goal is to find the heaviest weight possible for the prescribed number of repetitions. However, do not sacrifice technique for load.

233

LEVEL I
Back squat 3-x-5
Snatch 10 minutes practice
Walking lunge 3-x-20-meters

LEVEL II
Back squat 4-x-5
Establish 10RM power snatch
Overhead lunge 3-x-20-meters

LEVEL III
Back squat 5-x-5
Establish 10RM power snatch
Overhead lunge 4-x-20-meters

NOTES: All weights are determined by the strength of the individual. The goal is to find the heaviest weight possible for the prescribed number of repetitions. However, do not sacrifice technique for load.

WODs AT THE GYM

234

LEVEL I
1-minute cap:
20 snatch at 45 pounds (20.5 kg)/35 pounds (16 kg)
1-minute rest
3 minute cap:
20 snatch at 75 pounds (34 kg)/55 pounds (25 kg)
1-minute rest
5-minute cap:
20 snatch at 95 pounds (43 kg)/65 pounds (29.5 kg)

LEVEL II
1-minute cap:
30 snatch at 45 pounds (20.5 kg)/35 pounds (16 kg)
1-minute rest
3 minute cap:
30 snatch at 95 pounds (43 kg)/65 pounds (29.5 kg)
1-minute rest
5-minute cap:
30 snatch at 135 pounds (61 kg)/95 pounds (43 kg)

LEVEL III
1-minute cap:
30 snatch at 75 pounds (34 kg)/55 pounds (25 kg)
1-minute rest
3 minute cap:
30 snatch at 135 pounds (61 kg)/95 pounds (43 kg)
1-minute rest
5-minute cap:
30 snatch at 165 pounds (75 kg)/105 pounds (48 kg)

NOTES: At level I, focus on performing each rep perfectly. At level II and III athletes, attempt to perform large sets.

235

LEVEL I
5-minute AMRAP:
5 shoulder to overheads
10 deadlifts
15 box jumps

LEVEL II
2 rounds for total reps:
5-minute AMRAP:
5 shoulder to overheads (95 pounds [43 kg]/65 pounds [29.5 kg])
10 deadlifts (95 pounds [43 kg]/65 pounds [29.5 kg])
15 box jumps
Rest 5 minutes between rounds

LEVEL III
2 rounds for total reps:
5-minute AMRAP:
5 shoulder to overheads (135 pounds [61 kg]/95 pounds [43 kg])
10 deadlifts (135 pounds [61 kg]/95 pounds [43 kg])
15 box jumps
Rest 5 minutes between rounds

NOTES: This should be treated like a sprint. At level II and III, you get a 5-minutes recovery between 5-minute AMRAPs.

236

LEVEL I
10-minute AMRAP:
5 cleans (75 pounds
[34 kg]/55 pounds [25 kg])
10 situps
15 wall balls

LEVEL II
15-minute AMRAP:
5 cleans (95 pounds
[43 kg]/65 pounds [29.5 kg])
10 knees to elbows
15 wall balls

LEVEL III
20-minute AMRAP:
5 cleans (135 pounds
[61 kg]/95 pounds [43 kg])
10 toes to bar
15 wall balls

NOTES: Pick a moderate pace and try to maintain it. This is a marathon, not a sprint. For wall balls, men use a 20-pound (9 kg) ball to a 10-foot (3 m) target; women use a 14-pound (6.5 kg) ball to a 9-foot (2.7 m) target.

237

LEVEL I
10-minute AMRAP:
40 bar-facing burpees
10 overhead squats (65 pounds
[29.5 kg]/45 pounds [20.5 kg])
10 ring rows
10 pushups

LEVEL II
10-minute AMRAP:
50 bar-facing burpees
20 overhead squats (95 pounds
[43 kg]/65 pounds [29.5 kg])
5 muscle ups

LEVEL III
10-minute AMRAP:
60 bar-facing burpees
30 overhead squats (115 pounds
[52 kg]/75 pounds [34 kg])
10 muscle ups

NOTES: Bar-facing burpees require a two-footed jump over the bar between repetitions. Score is total reps completed.

238

LEVEL I
For time:
30 bench presses at ½ bodyweight
30 front squats at ½ bodyweight
30 shoulder to overheads at ½ bodyweight
30 deadlifts at ½ bodyweight

LEVEL II
For time:
30 bench presses at ¾ bodyweight
30 front squats at ¾ bodyweight
30 shoulder to overheads at ¾ bodyweight
30 deadlifts at ¾ bodyweight

LEVEL III
For time:
30 bench presses at bodyweight
30 front squats at bodyweight
30 shoulder to overheads at bodyweight
30 deadlifts at bodyweight

NOTES: If no benches are available, floor press can be substituted.

WODs AT THE GYM

239

LEVEL I
For time:
100-meter sled push
100-meter barbell carry (95 pounds [43 kg]/65 pounds [29.5 kg])
20 power snatches (95 pounds [43 kg]/65 pounds [29.5 kg])
20 power cleans (95 pounds [43 kg]/65 pounds [29.5 kg])

LEVEL II
For time:
100-meter sled push
100-meter barbell carry (115 pounds [52 kg]/75 pounds [34 kg])
20 power snatches (115 pounds [52 kg]/75 pounds [34 kg])
20 power cleans (115 pounds [52 kg]/75 pounds [34 kg])

LEVEL III
For time:
100-meter sled push
100-meter barbell carry (135 pounds [61 kg]/95 pounds [43 kg])
20 power snatches (135 pounds [61 kg]/95 pounds [43 kg])
20 power cleans (135 pounds [61 kg]/95 pounds [43 kg])

NOTES: Sled and barbell should start 100-meters apart. The weight loaded on the sled should correspond to the weight needed to complete the rest of the workout.

240

LEVEL I
2 rounds for time:
500-meter row
21 Russian-style kettlebell swings (35 pounds [16 kg]/25 pounds [11.5 kg])
15 burpees

LEVEL II
3 rounds for time:
500-meter row
21 American-style kettlebell swings (55 pounds [25 kg]/35 pounds [16 kg])
15 burpees

LEVEL III
3 rounds for time:
500-meter row
21 American-style kettlebell swings (70 pounds [32 kg]/50 pounds [22.5 kg])
15 burpees

NOTES: At level II and level III, attempt to complete the workout unbroken. At level I, focus on maintaining a steady pace throughout.

241

LEVEL I
10 rounds for time (65 pounds [29.5 kg]/45 pounds [20.5 kg]):
1 power snatch
1 oh squat
1 back squat thruster
1 oh squat

LEVEL II
12 rounds for time (75 pounds [34 kg]/55 pounds [25 kg]):
1 power snatch
1 oh squat
1 back squat thruster
1 oh squat

LEVEL III
15 rounds for time (95 pounds [43 kg]/65 pounds [29.5 kg]):
1 power snatch
1 oh squat
1 back squat thruster
1 oh squat

NOTE: Bar may only be dropped between completed rounds.

242

LEVEL I

For time:
30 wall balls
25 kettlebell swings
20 ring rows
15 pushups
10 wall walks

LEVEL II

For time:
40 wall balls
30 kettlebell swings
20 pullups
10 handstand pushups
5 muscle ups

LEVEL III

For time:
50 wall balls
40 kettlebell swings
30 pullups
20 handstand pushups
10 muscle ups

NOTES: At level II and level III, treat this workout like a sprint. If breaks are needed, they should be short and few. At level I, pace it much slower in an effort to manage your heart rate throughout. All kettlebell swings are American style.

243

LEVEL I

8-minute AMRAP:
1 rope climb to standing
3 power snatches (95 pounds [43 kg]/65 pounds [29.5 kg])
6 burpees over bar

LEVEL II

8-minute AMRAP:
1 rope climb
3 power snatches (135 pounds [61 kg]/95 pounds [43 kg])
6 burpees over bar

LEVEL III

8-minute AMRAP:
1 legless rope climb
3 squat snatches (135 pounds [61 kg]/95 pounds [43 kg])
6 burpees over bar

NOTES: At level I, pace this workout slowly and focus on technique during the snatches and climbs to standing. Level II and level III athletes shoud pick a faster pace and test your muscle endurance.

244

LEVEL I

2 rounds for time:
50-meter barbell overhead carry (45 pounds [20.5 kg]/35 pounds [16 kg])
20 situps
10 jumping pullups

LEVEL II

3 rounds for time:
100-meter barbell overhead carry (95 pounds [43 kg]/65 pounds [29.5 kg])
20 knees to elbows
10 pullups

LEVEL III

3 rounds for time:
100-meter barbell overhead carry (135 pounds [61 kg]/95 pounds [43 kg])
20 toes to bar
10 chest to bar pullups

NOTES: All levels should approach the overhead carry with a moderate pace, then attempt to do the remaining exercises unbroken, if possible.

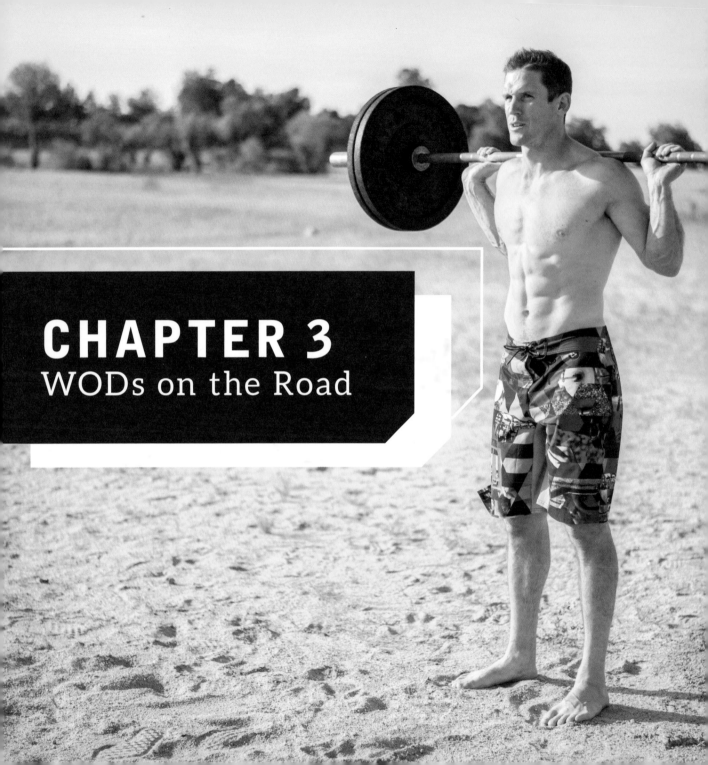

CHAPTER 3
WODs on the Road

This section is dedicated to workouts that can be done on the road, on vacation, or in a hotel gym. The idea here is to provide readers with a resource when they are out of town and away from their gym. This section is also a tool for those who don't enjoy the typical gym environment or simply cannot afford a monthly membership. Many of the following workouts require no equipment at all. Others require readers to possess portable implements like gymnastic rings, a refillable sandbag, or a jump rope. All WODs have been designed with the typical hotel gym in mind, so you won't find Olympic barbells or bumper plates here.

WODs ON THE ROAD

245

LEVEL I
2000-meter row for time

LEVEL II
2000-meter row for time

LEVEL III
2000-meter row for time

NOTES: Treat this like a four quarter race, with each 500-meters equaling one quarter. Do not sprint out of the gate and fail in the second quarter.

246

LEVEL I
2-mile (3.2 km) trail run

LEVEL II
4-mile (6.4 km) trail run

LEVEL III
5-mile (8 km) trail run

NOTE: Find a beautiful area and pick a moderate pace.

247

LEVEL I
5 burpees EMOTM; 20 minutes

LEVEL II
5 burpees + 1 muscle up EMOTM until failure to complete

LEVEL III
5 burpees + 3 muscle ups EMOTM until failure to complete

NOTES: At level I, if you fail before 20 minutes, rest the following minute and resume the workout.

248

LEVEL I
Bear crawl 200-meters for time

LEVEL II
Bear crawl 300-meters for time

LEVEL III
Bear crawl 400-meters for time

NOTES: Wear gloves to protect hands. Pick a moderate pace and try to stick to it. The fewer rests, the better.

249

LEVEL I
1-mile (1.6 km) sandbag carry

LEVEL II
2-mile (3.2 km) sandbag carry

LEVEL III
3-mile (4.8 km) sandbag carry

NOTES: This workout is all about completion. Carry the sandbag in any fashion; it may be loaded to any weight.

250

LEVEL I
10-minute AMRAP:
250-meter row
15 ring rows
10 burpees

LEVEL II
10-minute AMRAP:
250-meter row
15 pullups
10 burpees

LEVEL III
10-minute AMRAP:
250-meter row
15 pullups
10 burpees

NOTES: At level II and level III, attempt to complete all repetitions unbroken. At level I, practice managing the heart rate while continuing to progress through the workout.

WODs ON THE ROAD

251

LEVEL I
3-mile (4.8 km) run
Every mile (1.6 km) complete 30
air squats + 30 pushups

LEVEL II
4-mile (6.4 km) run
Every mile (1.6 km) complete 40
air squats + 40 pushups

LEVEL III
5-mile (8 km) run
Every mile (1.6 km) complete 50
air squats + 50 pushups

NOTES: Workout may be done outside
or on a treadmill. Each mile represents
a break from running but not a break
from the workout. Immediately begin
squats and pushups, then get right back
on the run.

252

LEVEL I
5-minute AMRAP:
5 stone squats
10 ring rows

LEVEL II
5-minute AMRAP:
5 stone squats
5 ring pullups

LEVEL III
5-minute AMRAP:
5 stone squats
5 muscle ups

NOTES: Any stone will do. Rings
can be hung from a tree branch or
any solid structure to desired height.
This workout is meant to be a sprint,
so go at it hard.

253

LEVEL I
EMOTM; 10-minutes:
30 single unders
5 pushups

LEVEL II
EMOTM; 10-minutes:
20 double unders
5 piked pushups

LEVEL III
EMOTM; 10-minutes:
30 double unders
5 handstand pushups

NOTES: This is a skill test. At level
II and level III, attempt to complete
unbroken.

254

LEVEL I
10-minute AMRAP:
5 ring rows
50 single unders
100-meter car push

LEVEL II
15-minute AMRAP:
5 ring pull ups
25 double unders
100-meter car push

LEVEL III
20-minute AMRAP:
5 muscle ups
50 double unders
100-meter car push

NOTES: Find a level stretch of road with trees nearby. If such a location does not exist, substitute handstand holds for muscle ups and pushups for ring rows.

255

LEVEL I
EMOTM; 10-minutes:
7 ring rows
7 hollow rocks

LEVEL II
EMOTM; 10-minutes:
1 muscle up
7 candlestick to deck squats

LEVEL III
EMOTM; 10-minutes:
3 muscle ups
7 candlestick to deck squats

NOTES: At level II and level III, athletes must candlestick (lift hips and point toes toward ceiling) before rolling into your deck squats.

256

LEVEL I
1-minute on/1-minute off rowing intervals for 10 intervals
Score is max distance

LEVEL II
1-minute on/1-minute off rowing intervals for 10 intervals
Score is max distance

LEVEL III
1-minute on/1-minute off rowing intervals for 10 intervals
Score is max distance

WODs ON THE ROAD

257

LEVEL I
6 rounds for time:
5 ring rows
10 pushups
15 air squats

LEVEL II
8 rounds for time:
5 ring pullups
10 pushups
15 air squats

LEVEL III
10 rounds for time:
5 muscle ups
10 ring dips
15 air squats

NOTES: This workout tests muscle endurance. Attempt to complete as much of it unbroken as possible, but if forced to rest, keep rest periods short.

258

LEVEL I
2 rounds for time:
400-meter farmer's carry
25 pushups

LEVEL II
3 rounds for time:
400-meter farmer's carry
25 piked pushups

LEVEL III
3 rounds for time:
400-meter farmer's carry
25 handstand pushups

NOTES: Farmer's carry can be any weight. Dumbbells will work best. At level II, use a bench for the knees to complete the piked pushups.

259

LEVEL I
EMOTM; 10-minutes:
5 jumping pullups
5 pushups

LEVEL II
EMOTM; 10-minutes:
1 muscle up
5 piked pushups

LEVEL III
EMOTM; 10-minutes:
4 muscle ups
4 handstand pushups

NOTES: This is a skill test. All exercises should be completed unbroken, if possible.

260

LEVEL I
5 rounds for completion:
200-meter uphill treadmill run
(5 percent grade)
400-meter flat treadmill run

LEVEL II
7 rounds for completion:
200-meter uphill treadmill run
(10 percent grade)
400-meter flat treadmill run

LEVEL III
10 rounds for completion:
200-meter uphill treadmill run
(15 percent grade)
400-meter flat treadmill run

NOTES: Slow and steady wins the race on the uphill climbs. Let the legs out on the flat runs.

261

LEVEL I
Accumulate 5 minutes in a plank
Accumulate 4 minutes in a V sit
Accumulate 3 minutes in a wall handstand
Accumulate 2-minute in a hip bridge
Accumulate 1-minute in dip support

LEVEL II
Accumulate 5 minutes in a plank
Accumulate 4 minutes in an L sit
Accumulate 3 minutes in a free handstand
Accumulate 2-minute in a bridge
Accumulate 1-minute in dip support

LEVEL III
Accumulate 5 minutes in a plank
Accumulate 4 minutes in an L sit
Accumulate 3 minutes in a free handstand
Accumulate 2-minute in a bridge
Accumulate 1-minute in dip support

NOTES: You can mix and match these sets any way you choose. Keep a running track of everything and attempt to complete everything in less than 30 minutes.

262

LEVEL I
Complete the following sets of single unders unbroken for time:
5-10-15-20-25-30-35-40-45-50-45-40-35-30-25-20-15-10-5

LEVEL II
Complete the following sets of double unders unbroken for time:
5-10-15-20-25-30-35-40-45-50-45-40-35-30-25-20-15-10-5

LEVEL III
Complete the following sets of double unders unbroken for time:
5-10-15-20-25-30-35-40-45-50-45-40-35-30-25-20-15-10-5

NOTE: If a set is failed midway through, start that set over again.

WODs ON THE ROAD

263

LEVEL I

In 15 minutes accumulate as much mileage as possible using the rower and treadmill

Max distance on either interval is 800-meters

LEVEL II

In 20 minutes accumulate as much mileage as possible using the rower and treadmill

Max distance on either interval is 800-meters

LEVEL III

In 30 minutes accumulate as much mileage as possible using the rower and treadmill

Max distance on either interval is 800-meters

264

LEVEL I

EMOTM; 10-minutes:
5 burpees
5 knees to elbows

LEVEL II

EMOTM; 10-minutes:
1 muscle up
5 toes to rings

LEVEL III

EMOTM; 10-minutes:
4 muscle ups
5 toes to rings

NOTES: This is a skill test. All repetitions should be completed unbroken.

265

LEVEL I

5000-meter row for time

LEVEL II

5000-meter row for time

LEVEL III

5000-meter row for time

266

LEVEL I
10-minute AMRAP:
20 squats
15 jumping dips
10 pushups

LEVEL II
15-minute AMRAP:
20 squat jumps
15 bar dips
10 piked pushups

LEVEL III
20-minute AMRAP:
20 squat jumps
15 ring dips
10 handstand pushups

NOTES: Squat jumps do not need to be maximum height. Ring dips and handstand pushups may be kipped if necessary.

267

LEVEL I
For time:
1000-meter row
30 ball slams
30 dumbbell swings
30 abmat situps
30 wall balls
1000-meter row

LEVEL II
For time:
1600-meter row
40 ball slams
40 dumbbell swings
40 abmat situps
40 wall balls
1600-meter row

LEVEL III
For time:
2000-meter row
50 ball slams
50 dumbbell swings
50 abmat situps
50 wall balls
2000-meter row

NOTES: At level I, do Russian-style swings (eye level); At level II and level III, do American-style swings (overhead). Any weight medicine ball will work for ball slams and wall balls. Height of target should be 10 feet (3 m) for men and 9 feet (2.7 m) for women.

WODs ON THE ROAD

268

LEVEL I
6 rounds for time:
5 jumping ring pullups
10 air squats

LEVEL II
8 rounds for time:
2 muscle ups
4 deck squats

LEVEL III
10 rounds for time:
4 muscle ups
8 deck squats

NOTES: This is meant to be a sprint, so attack the workout. you need to know your ability level for muscle ups.

269

LEVEL I
7-minute AMRAP:
250-meter row
10 dumbbell swings
10 burpees

LEVEL II
7-minute AMRAP:
250-meter row
10 dumbbell swings
10 burpees

LEVEL III
7-minute AMRAP:
250-meter row
10 dumbbell swings
10 burpees

NOTES: At level I, do Russian-style swings (eye level); At level II and level III, do American-style swings (overhead). This is a fast workout but not a sprint.

270

LEVEL I
EMOTM; 12-minutes:
5 burpees
5 Dumbbell push presses each arm

LEVEL II
EMOTM; 12-minutes:
5 burpees
5 Dumbbell snatches each arm

LEVEL III
EMOTM; 12-minutes:
10 burpees
5 Dumbbell snatches each arm

NOTES: Dumbbell snatches must touch the ground between reps. Complete 5 repetitions on the right arm before switching to the left.

271

LEVEL I
For time:
50 wall balls
25 jumping pullups
25 pushups

LEVEL II
For time:
75 wall balls
50 pullups
50 piked pushups

LEVEL III
For time:
100 wall balls
50 pullups
50 handstand pushups

NOTES: Any weight medicine ball will work for wall balls. Height of target should be 10 feet (3 m) for men and 9 feet (2.7 m) for women. Pullups can be done on a bar or tree limb. Handstand pushups can be kipped and should be done on a wall or tree trunk. Piked pushups should be done with knees on a bench or a ledge.

272

LEVEL I
EMOTM; 10-minutes:
6 air squats
3 knees to elbows

LEVEL II
EMOTM; 10-minutes:
6 deck squats
3 toes to rings

LEVEL III
EMOTM; 10-minutes:
6 alternating pistols
3 skin the cats

NOTES: This is a skill test and should be completed unbroken if possible. A skin the cat is completed when the hips are passed through the rings in a backward tuck while holding onto the rings. Once the hips pass below the level of the head, return the hips and legs to the starting position under the rings.

273

LEVEL I
3 rounds for time:
200-meter medicine ball carry
10 burpee wall balls

LEVEL II
3 rounds for time:
400-meter medicine ball carry
15 burpee wall balls

LEVEL III
3 rounds for time:
400-meter medicine ball carry
20 burpee wall balls

NOTES: Any weight medicine ball will work for wall balls. Target should be 10 feet (3 m) for men and 9 feet (2.7 m) for women. The chest must touch the ball for each burpee to count.

WODs ON THE ROAD

274

LEVEL I
As far as possible in 7-minutes:
1 to 10 ring rows
20 to 200 single unders

LEVEL II
As far as possible in 7-minutes:
1 to 10 pullups
10 to 100 double unders

LEVEL III
As far as possible in 7-minutes:
1 to 10 muscle ups
10 to 100 double unders

NOTES: Pullups can be done on a bar or rings, depending on location. Alternate between sets of muscle ups/pullups/ring rows and the jump rope. The score for the workout is the total number of repetitions.

275

LEVEL I
10-minute AMRAP:
20 dumbbell swings
6-x-20-meter shuttle run
Must carry dumbbell during shuttle

LEVEL II
15-minute AMRAP:
20 dumbbell swings
6-x-20-meter shuttle run
Must carry dumbbell during shuttle

LEVEL III
20-minute AMRAP:
20 dumbbell swings
6-x-20-meter shuttle run
Must carry dumbbell during shuttle

NOTES: Dumbbells can be any weight. At level I, do Russian-style swings (eye level); At level II and level III, do American-style swings (overhead). Dumbbell can be carried in any fashion.

276

LEVEL I
Complete 8 x :20 rounds for each exercise:
Ring rows
Burpees
Wall walks
Air squats

LEVEL II
Complete 8 x :20 rounds for each exercise:
Pullups
Burpees
Handstand walk
Deck squats

LEVEL III
Complete 8 x :20 rounds for each exercise:
Muscle ups
Burpees
Handstand walk
Deck squats

NOTES: Rest exactly :10 between rounds. Only after compleating 8 rounds of each exercise may you move on to the next exercise.

277

LEVEL I
EMOTM; until failure to complete:
100-meter treadmill run

LEVEL II
EMOTM; until failure to complete:
100-meter treadmill run
Every round add ½ degree of incline

LEVEL III
EMOTM; until failure to complete:
100-meter treadmill run
Every round add 1 degree of incline

NOTES: Set the speed of the treadmill to any speed they choose. The workout is over when they can no longer complete the 100-meters in the time allotted.

278 (CINDY)

LEVEL I
20-minute AMRAP:
5 ring rows
10 pushups
15 air squats

LEVEL II
20-minute AMRAP:
5 pullups
10 pushups
15 air squats

LEVEL III
20-minute AMRAP:
5 pullups
10 pushups
15 air squats

NOTES: This is a popular benchmark known as "Cindy." At level II and level III, move as quickly as possible between exercises. At level I, maintain a moderate pace and ensure quality repetitions.

279

LEVEL I
7-minute AMRAP burpees

LEVEL II
7-minute AMRAP burpee pullups

LEVEL III
7-minute AMRAP burpee muscle ups

NOTES: At level II and level III, rings and pullup bars should be a minimum of 6 inches (15 cm) above your reach.

WODs ON THE ROAD

280

LEVEL I
3 rounds for completion:
5 stone deadlifts
400-meter run

LEVEL II
4 rounds for completion:
5 stone deadlifts
400-meter run

LEVEL III
5 rounds for completion:
5 stone deadlifts
400-meter run

NOTES: Any stone will work for this workout. Be creative and find something that is both challenging to lift and challenging to grip.

281

LEVEL I
5-x-400-meter treadmill hill sprints (5 percent grade)
Rest 3 minutes between efforts

LEVEL II
5-x-400-meter treadmill hill sprints (8 percent grade)
Rest 2 minutes between efforts

LEVEL III
5-x-400-meter treadmill hill sprints (10 percent grade)
Rest 1-minute between efforts

NOTES: Adjust speed of treadmill as needed during sprints. These may not be much of a "sprint."

282

LEVEL I
3 rounds for time:
3 rope climb to standing
10 hand release pushups

LEVEL II
5 rounds for time:
1 rope climb
10 piked pushups

LEVEL III
5 rounds for time:
1 legless rope climb
10 handstand pushups

NOTES: Complete this workout if you have access to a rope. Rope climbs to standing should begin on the back and finish upright using only the arms.

283

LEVEL I
2-mile (3.2 km) object carry for time

LEVEL II
3-mile (4.8 km) object carry for time

LEVEL III
4-mile (6.4 km) object carry for time

NOTES: Any object will do. Dumbbells and medicine balls are most common, but stones and branches work just as well. Pick a slow pace and remain steady.

284

LEVEL I
12-minute AMRAP:
30 situps
¼-mile (400 m) sandbag carry

LEVEL II
12-minute AMRAP:
30 knees to elbows
¼-mile (400 m) sandbag carry

LEVEL III
12-minute AMRAP:
30 toes to rings
½-mile (800 m) sandbag carry

NOTES: Sandbag can be filled to any weight. This is more of a for-time workout, but if you finish fast begin toes to rings right away.

285

LEVEL I
For time:
200-meter overhead object carry

LEVEL II
For time:
300-meter overhead object carry

LEVEL III
For time:
400-meter overhead object carry

NOTES: Any object will work if it is 40 pounds (18 kg) or more for men and 30 pounds (13.5 kg) or more for women. Do not rest the object on your head.

286

LEVEL I
3 rounds for completion:
5 ring swings
5 pushups
5 knees to elbows
5 air squats

LEVEL II
4 rounds for completion:
5 ring swings
5 ring dips
5 toes to rings
5 air squats

LEVEL III
5 rounds for completion:
5 ring swings
5 ring dips
5 toes to rings
5 pistol squats

NOTES: Rings must be hung high and secure to accommodate swinging. At level II and level III, you will need to muscle up to complete the dip portion.

287

LEVEL I
EMOTM; 10-minutes:
1 situp + pushup
3 jumping ring pullups
5 knees to elbows

LEVEL II
EMOTM; 15-minutes:
1 ring muscle up
3 ring pullups
5 toes to rings

LEVEL III
EMOTM; 20-minutes:
1 ring muscle up
3 ring pullups
5 toes to rings

NOTES: Attempt to complete the complex without dropping off the rings.

288

LEVEL I
For time:
500-meter row buy in
3 rounds:
30 unbroken single unders
10 burpees
10 situps
500-meter buy out

LEVEL II
For time:
500-meter row buy in
4 rounds:
30 double unders
10 burpees
10 situps
500-meter buy out

LEVEL III
For time:
500-meter row buy in
5 rounds:
30 unbroken double unders
10 burpees
10 situps
500-meter buy out

NOTES: The 500-meter row buys into the 3/4/5 round workout. It also is the final piece to complete it.

289

LEVEL I
3 rounds for time:
10 Dumbbell push presses
10 Dumbbell deadlifts
10 Dumbbell burpees

LEVEL II
4 rounds for time:
10 Dumbbell push presses
10 Dumbbell deadlifts
10 Dumbbell burpees

LEVEL III
5 rounds for time:
10 Dumbbell push presses
10 Dumbbell deadlifts
10 Dumbbell burpees

NOTES: Dumbbells can be any weight. For the burpee portion the dumbbells must remain in the athlete's hands throughout the burpee motion. No clap is necessary at the top, just a press. Deadlifts must touch the ground during each repetition.

290

LEVEL I
10-minute AMRAP:
100-meter treadmill sprint
20 walking lunges
10 pushups
10 air squats

LEVEL II
12-minute AMRAP:
200-meter treadmill sprint
30 walking lunges
20 pushups
10 deck squats

LEVEL III
15-minute AMRAP:
200-meter treadmill sprint
30 walking lunges
20 clapping pushups
10 deck squats

NOTES: This is a higher volume workout, requiring you to break up sets, if necessary. Keep rest periods short and few.

291

LEVEL I
21-15-9 for time:
Jumping pullup
Pushup
Air squat

LEVEL II
15-12-9-6-3 for time:
Pullup
Piked pushup
Assisted pistol squat

LEVEL III
21-18-15-12-9-6-3 for time:
Strict pullup
Strict handstand pushup
Pistol squat

NOTES: At level III, there is a high degree of difficulty. Strict pullups and handstand pushups are required. At level II, assist pistol squats by rolling up through the squat or by using a post.

WODs ON THE ROAD

292

LEVEL I

For time:
20 dumbbell ground to overheads
20 dumbbell swings
20 dumbbell front squats

LEVEL II

2 rounds for time:
20 dumbbell ground to overheads
20 dumbbell swings
20 dumbbell front squats

LEVEL III

3 rounds for time:
20 dumbbell ground to overheads
20 dumbbell swings
20 dumbbell front squats

NOTES: Ground to overheads can be done in any fashion (snatch, clean and jerk, etc.). At level I, do Russian-style swings (eye level); At level II and level III, do American-style swings (overhead). Dumbbells can be any weight.

293

LEVEL I

200-meter dumbbell farmer's carry
Every 50-meters perform 5 thrusters

LEVEL II

300-meter dumbbell farmer's carry
Every 50-meters perform 8 thrusters

LEVEL III

400-meter dumbbell farmer's carry
Every 50-meters perform 10 thrusters

NOTES: Dumbbells do not need to be heavy. The goal is to complete the workout in 30 minutes.

294

LEVEL I

1-mile (1.6 km) uphill walk on treadmill (15 percent grade)

LEVEL II

1.5-mile (2.4 km) uphill walk on treadmill (15 percent grade)

LEVEL III

2-mile (3.2 km) uphill walk on treadmill (15 percent grade)

NOTES: This is for completion, so don't be in a rush. Try to maintain a steady pace the entire time.

295

LEVEL I
2 rounds for time:
100-meter dumbbell waiter's walk
10 single arm dumbbell thrusters
6 single arm burpees

LEVEL II
3 rounds for time:
100-meter dumbbell waiter's walk
10 single arm dumbbell thrusters
6 single arm burpees

LEVEL III
3 rounds for time:
100-meter dumbbell waiter's walk
15 single arm dumbbell thrusters
10 single arm burpees

NOTES: Waiter's walk is a single-arm overhead carry. Alternate arms as needed on all exercises.

296

LEVEL I
Dumbbell overhead press 3-x-5
Dumbbell step up 3-x-5
Chinup 3-x-5
Hanging L sit hold 3 × :10

LEVEL II
Dumbbell overhead press 4-x-5
Dumbbell step up 4-x-5
Weighted chinup 4-x-5
Hanging L sit hold 3 × :20

LEVEL III
Dumbbell overhead press 5-x-5
Dumbbell step up 5-x-5
Weighted chinup 5-x-5
Hanging L sit hold 3 × :30

NOTES: Dumbbell weights should be adjusted throughout the workout. The goal is to find the heaviest weight with which you can successfully perform each exercise.

297

LEVEL I
Dumbbell bench press 3-x-5
Dumbbell front squat 3-x-10
Dumbbell row 3-x-10
Dumbbell Russian twist 3-x-20

LEVEL II
Dumbbell bench press 4-x-5
Dumbbell front squat 4-x-10
Dumbbell row 4-x-10
Dumbbell Russian twist 3-x-20

LEVEL III
Dumbbell bench press 5-x-5
Dumbbell front squat 5-x-10
Dumbbell row 5-x-10
Dumbbell Russian twist 3-x-20

NOTES: Dumbbell weights should be adjusted throughout the workout. The goal is to find the heaviest weight with which you can successfully perform each exercise.

298

LEVEL I

10-minute AMRAP:
5 single arm dumbbell front squats
5 single arm dumbbell swings
5 single arm dumbbell deadlifts
50 single unders

LEVEL II

15-minute AMRAP:
5 single arm dumbbell overhead squats
5 single arm dumbbell swings
5 single arm dumbbell deadlifts
30 double unders

LEVEL III

20-minute AMRAP:
5 single arm dumbbell overhead squats
5 single arm dumbbell swings
5 single arm dumbbell deadlifts
50 double unders

NOTES: Dumbbells can be any weight. Alternate arms as necessary on all exercises. Dumbbell swings should be American-style.

299

LEVEL I

6-minute AMRAP:
5 dumbbell thrusters
10-meter dumbbell bear crawl

LEVEL II

8-minute AMRAP:
5 dumbbell thrusters
10-meter dumbbell bear crawl

LEVEL III

10-minute AMRAP:
5 dumbbell thrusters
10-meter dumbbell bear crawl

NOTES: Dumbbells can be any weight. For bear crawl, dumbbells must move with hands for the entire 10-meters.

300

LEVEL I

For time:
1000-meter row
1-mile (1.6 km) treadmill run on 2 percent grade
1000-meter row

LEVEL II

For time:
1500-meter row
1-mile (1.6 km) treadmill run on 3 percent grade
1500-meter row

LEVEL III

For time:
2000-meter row
1-mile (1.6 km) treadmill run on 4 percent grade
2000-meter row

NOTES: This is an aerobic endurance workout. Pick a steady pace and stick to it.

301

LEVEL I
EMOTM; 10-minutes:
5 jumping pullups
30 single unders

LEVEL II
EMOTM; 10-minutes:
5 pullups
15 double unders

LEVEL III
EMOTM; 15-minutes:
5 strict pullups
25 double unders

NOTES: If you fail to complete a round in the minute, rest the following minute and then resume.

302

LEVEL I
8-minute AMRAP:
5 dumbbell hang cleans
7 dumbbell shoulder to overheads
9 dumbbell deadlifts

LEVEL II
10-minute AMRAP:
5 dumbbell hang cleans
7 dumbbell shoulder to overheads
9 dumbbell deadlifts

LEVEL III
12-minute AMRAP:
5 dumbbell hang cleans
7 dumbbell shoulder to overheads
9 dumbbell deadlifts

NOTES: At level II and level III, choose dumbbells so that at least one round of the workout can be completed unbroken. At level I, keep the weight light.

303

LEVEL I
12-minute AMRAP:
4 dumbbell front squats
8 jumping pullups

LEVEL II
12-minute AMRAP:
4 dumbbell front squats
8 pullups

LEVEL III
16-minute AMRAP:
4 dumbbell front squats
8 strict pullups

NOTES: This is a high-volume workout, so there is no need to sprint initially. Dumbbells should be heavy to simulate a difficult front squat. Goal is to complete 10 rounds.

WODs ON THE ROAD

304

LEVEL I
3 rounds for time:
10 pushups
20 burpees
60 single unders

LEVEL II
4 rounds for time:
10 bar dips
20 burpees
30 double unders

LEVEL III
5 rounds for time:
10 ring dips
20 burpees
30 double unders

NOTE: Athletes should do this unbroken, if possible.

305

LEVEL I
4 rounds for time:
50-meter dumbbell farmer's carry
5 jumping pullups
10 pushups
15 air squats

LEVEL II
4 rounds for time:
75-meter dumbbell farmer's carry
5 pullups
10 pushups
15 dumbbell front squats

LEVEL III
4 rounds for time:
100-meter dumbbell farmer's carry
5 strict pullups
10 pushups
15 dumbbell front squats

NOTES: Dumbbells can be any weight. If no outdoor area is available for farmer's carry, it may be done on the treadmill at a walking pace.

306

LEVEL I
500 single unders for time
Every mistake complete 5 pushups

LEVEL II
250 double unders for time
Every mistake complete 10 pushups

LEVEL III
500 double unders for time
Every mistake complete 10 pushups

NOTE: Record number of attempts required to reach goal.

307

LEVEL I

6-minute AMRAP:
3 dumbbell thrusters
3 jumping pullups
6 dumbbell thrusters
6 jumping pullups
9 dumbbell thrusters
9 jumping pullups
(and so forth)

LEVEL II

8-minute AMRAP:
3 dumbbell thrusters
3 pullups
6 dumbbell thrusters
6 pullups
9 dumbbell thrusters
9 pullups
(and so forth)

LEVEL III

10-minute AMRAP:
3 dumbbell thrusters
3 pullups
6 dumbbell thrusters
6 pullups
9 dumbbell thrusters
9 pullups
(and so forth)

NOTES: Continue up the repetition ladder until time expires. At level I, focus on form over speed.

308

LEVEL I

3 rounds for time:
15 pushups
10 situps
5 jumping ring dips

LEVEL II

4 rounds for time:
15 pushups
10 toes to rings
5 ring dips

LEVEL III

5 rounds for time:
15 pushups
10 toes to rings
5 ring dips

NOTES: At level III, you will have to muscle up in order to complete their ring dips. At level II, you can use assistance to reach rings.

WODs ON THE ROAD

309

LEVEL I
15-minute cap:
40 burpees
10 dumbbell snatches
30 burpees
10 dumbbell snatches
20 burpees
10 dumbbell snatches
10 burpees
AMRAP dumbbell snatches

LEVEL II
15-minute cap:
40 burpees
20 dumbbell snatches
30 burpees
20 dumbbell snatches
20 burpees
20 dumbbell snatches
10 burpees
AMRAP dumbbell snatches

LEVEL III
15-minute cap:
40 burpees
30 dumbbell snatches
30 burpees
30 dumbbell snatches
20 burpees
30 dumbbell snatches
10 burpees
AMRAP dumbbell snatches

NOTES: Dumbbell snatches should be taken from the ground to overhead in one continuous movement. Alternate arms each repetition.

310

LEVEL I
10-minute AMRAP:
9 dumbbell deadlifts
12 pushups
15 step ups
200-meter treadmill sprint

LEVEL II
10-minute AMRAP:
9 dumbbell deadlifts
12 pushups
15 box jumps
200-meter treadmill sprint

LEVEL III
10-minute AMRAP:
9 dumbbell deadlifts
12 clapping pushups
15 box jumps
200-meter treadmill sprint

NOTES: Dumbbells should touch the ground outside the feet between each deadlift rep. A bench can be used for box jumps and step ups.

311

LEVEL I
Run 1-mile (1.6 km) with a medicine ball
Every 200-meters complete 10 front squats

LEVEL II
Run 1.5-miles (2.4 km) with a medicine ball
Every 200-meters complete 10 front squats

LEVEL III
Run 2-miles (3.2 km) with a medicine ball
Every 200-meters, complete 10 front squats

NOTES: Medicine ball can be carried in any fashion. Front squats should be done with ball in front of the face. If no medicine ball is available, a dumbbell may be substituted.

312

LEVEL I
Ride 10 miles (16 km) on stationary bike for time
Every 5 minutes complete:
5 jumping pullups
10 pushups
15 squats

LEVEL II
Ride 15-miles (24 km) on stationary bike for time
Every 5 minutes complete:
5 pullups
10 pushups
15 squats

LEVEL III
Ride 20 miles (32 km) on stationary bike for time
Every 5 minutes complete:
5 pullups
10 handstand pushups
15 pistol squats

NOTE: No additional rest should be taken while transitioning between bike and calisthenics.

WODs ON THE ROAD

313

LEVEL I
EMOTM; 10-minutes:
1 situp
1 burpee
2 situps
2 burpees
3 situps
3 burpees
(and so forth)

LEVEL II
EMOTM; 10-minutes:
1 knee to elbow
1 burpee
2 knees to elbows
2 burpees
3 knees to elbows
3 burpees
(and so forth)

LEVEL III
EMOTM; 10-minutes:
1 toes to bar
1 burpee
2 toes to bar
2 burpees
3 toes to bar
3 burpees
(and so forth)

NOTES: Continue until failure to complete the prescribed number of reps or until 10 minutes has elapsed.

314

LEVEL I
EMOTM; 10-minutes:
5 pushups
5 hollow rocks

LEVEL II
EMOTM; 15-minutes:
5 bar dips
5 situps

LEVEL III
EMOTM; 20-minutes:
5 ring dips
5 V ups

NOTES: If you fail to complete the required work in the minute, rest 1 round and then resume.

315

LEVEL I
21-15-9
Singe unders
Burpees
Air squats

LEVEL II
21-15-9
Double unders
Burpees
Deck squats

LEVEL III
21-15-9
Double unders
Burpees
Deck squats

NOTES: This is meant to be a sprint, so pick a fast pace and don't worry about burning out. At level III, not use hands to assist deck squats, but level II athletes can.

316

LEVEL I
10-minute AMRAP:
10 dumbbell swings
15-meter bear crawl
20 steps high knees

LEVEL II
12-minute AMRAP:
10 dumbbell swings
15-meter bear crawl
20 steps high knees

LEVEL III
15-minute AMRAP:
10 dumbbell swings
15-meter bear crawl
20 steps high knees

NOTES: At level I, dumbbell swings should be performed to eye level and to vertical for level II and level III athletes. Pacing is important on this workout, so don't go out too fast.

317

LEVEL I
10-minute AMRAP:
10 jumping pullups
30 air squats

LEVEL II
10-minute AMRAP:
10 pullups
15 alternating pistol squats

LEVEL III
10-minute AMRAP:
10 strict pullups
30 alternating pistol squats

NOTES: At level II, you may use assistance to complete pistol squats, either in the form of a roll to stand or by using a post to support themselves.

318

LEVEL I
For time:
10 down to 1 dumbbell push press
1 up to 10 pushup

LEVEL II
For time:
10 down to 1 dumbbell push press
1 up to 10 single arm pushup from knees

LEVEL III
For time:
10 down to 1 dumbbell push press
1 up to 10 single arm pushup

NOTES: Dumbbells should be a weight that is challenging to complete 10 consecutive repetitions.

319

LEVEL I
For time:
1000-meter row
30 hollow rocks
15 burpees
30 hollow rocks
1000-meter row

LEVEL II
For time:
1000-meter row
40 hollow rocks
20 burpees
40 hollow rocks
1000-meter row

LEVEL III
For time:
1000-meter row
50 hollow rocks
25 burpees
50 hollow rocks
1000-meter row

320

LEVEL I
3-x-1-minute rounds:
Dead hang hold
Plank hold
Downward dog hold
Wall squat hold

LEVEL II
4-x-1-minute rounds:
Dead hang hold
Plank hold
Wall handstand hold
Air squat hold

LEVEL III
5-x-1-minute rounds:
Dead hang hold
Plank hold
Wall handstand hold
Air squat hold

NOTES: Wall squats must be done just below parallel. Dead hangs should be with straight arms. Planks are on the elbows.

321

LEVEL I
8-minute AMRAP:
100-meter treadmill run on incline
10
10 dumbbell front squats
10 pushups

LEVEL II
10-minute AMRAP:
100-meter treadmill run on incline
12
10 dumbbell hang squat cleans
10 piked pushups

LEVEL III
12-minute AMRAP:
100-meter treadmill run on incline
15
10 dumbbell hang squat cleans
10 handstand pushups

NOTES: The treadmill run can be a run, jog, or walk, depending on ability. Piked pushups should be done with feet or knees resting on a bench and torso as close to vertical as possible. Dumbbells should be difficult to complete 10 consecutive repetitions.

322

LEVEL I
Tabata row for meters

LEVEL II
Tabata row for meters

LEVEL III
Tabata row for meters

NOTES: You may adjust the damper to the setting you prefer. Complete 8 intervals of 20 seconds rowing and 10 seconds resting. Score is the total meters traveled.

323

LEVEL I
For time:
1-mile (1.6 km) dumbbell carry on treadmill incline 10 (20 pounds [9 kg]/10 pounds [4.5 kg])

LEVEL II
2-mile (3.2 km) dumbbell carry on treadmill incline 12 (30 pounds [13.5 kg]/20 pounds [9 kg])

LEVEL III
3-mile (4.8 km) dumbbell carry on treadmill incline 15 (40 pounds [18 kg]/30 pounds [13.5 kg])

NOTES: Dumbbell can be carried in any fashion but may not be set down until distance is complete. This is a mentally challenging workout, so be prepared!

324

LEVEL I
EMOTM; 20-minutes:
1 dumbbell plank row
1 dumbbell burpee

LEVEL II
EMOTM; 20-minutes:
2 dumbbell plank rows
2 dumbbell burpees

LEVEL III
EMOTM; 20-minutes:
3 dumbbell plank rows
3 dumbbell burpees

NOTES: Dumbbell plank rows are counted as 1, 2, or 3 reps each arm. Dumbbells can be any weight.

WODs ON THE ROAD

325

LEVEL I
For time:
300-meter row
10 air squats
250-meter row
20 air squats
200-meter row
30 air squats
150-meter row
40 air squats
100-meter row
50 air squats

LEVEL II
For time:
500-meter row
10 air squats
400-meter row
20 air squats
300-meter row
30 air squats
200-meter row
40 air squats
100-meter row
50 air squats

LEVEL III
For time:
500-meter row
10 jump squats
400-meter row
20 jump squats
300-meter row
30 jump squats
200-meter row
40 jump squats
100-meter row
50 jump squats

NOTES: At level III, show air beneath your feet during jump squats, it doesn't matter how much. Monitor depth closely because fatigue will lead to shallow squats.

326

LEVEL I
For time:
10 down to 1 dumbbell hang clean and press
2 up to 20 situps

LEVEL II
For time:
10 down to 1 dumbbell hang clean and press
2 up to 20 knees to elbows

LEVEL III
For time:
10 down to 1 dumbbell hang clean and press
2 up to 20 toes to bar

NOTES: Clean and presses should start in the hang position and be swung up to shoulders before pressing overhead. Situps should be done with straight legs.

327

LEVEL I
E2MOTM 20-minutes:
¼-mile (400 m) stationary bike sprint
5 jumping pullups
10 pushups
15 air squats

LEVEL II
E2MOTM 24 minutes:
¼-mile (400 m) stationary bike sprint
5 pullups
10 pushups
15 air squats

LEVEL III
E2MOTM 30-minutes:
¼-mile (400 m) stationary bike sprint
5 strict pullups
10 pushups
15 air squats

NOTES: At level I and level II, you may do pushups from knees; at level III, you may not. Each round must restart every 2 minutes. If a round is finished after time, you must sit out the next round before resuming.

328

LEVEL I
Climb 50 flights of stairs for time

LEVEL II
Climb 75 flights of stairs for time

LEVEL III
Climb 100 flights of stairs for time

NOTES: Stairs can be climbed on a stair mill or in a hotel stairwell. Flights must be repeated if hotel is not tall enough to complete. Flights should also be walked down rather than taking the elevator

WODs ON THE ROAD

329

LEVEL I
10-minute AMRAP:
50-meter suitcase carry left hand
50-meter suitcase carry right hand
10 air squats

LEVEL II
15-minute AMRAP:
75-meter suitcase carry left hand
75-meter suitcase carry right hand
10 suitcase overhead squats

LEVEL III
20-minute AMRAP:
100-meter suitcase carry left hand
100-meter suitcase carry right hand
10 suitcase overhead squats

NOTES: Suitcase should be loaded to 50+ pounds (22.5 kg) for level III, 40+ pounds (18 kg) for level II, and 30+ pounds (13.5 kg) for level I. Bonus points for doing it in the airport.

330

LEVEL I
6-minute AMRAP:
10 Dumbbell step ups
10 Dumbbell burpees
Rest 4 minutes
6-minute AMRAP:
5 dumbbell thrusters
5 jumping pullups

LEVEL II
8-minute AMRAP:
10 Dumbbell step ups
10 Dumbbell burpees
Rest 3 minutes
8-minute AMRAP:
5 dumbbell thrusters
5 pullups

LEVEL III
10-minute AMRAP:
10 Dumbbell step ups
10 Dumbbell burpees
Rest 2 minutes
10-minute AMRAP:
5 dumbbell thrusters
5 strict pullups

NOTES: Dumbbells can be scaled to any weight. Step ups should be done on a bench or box.

331

LEVEL I
4 rounds for time:
8 situps
8 burpees to target
8 single arm dumbbell front squats

LEVEL II
6 rounds for time:
8 knees to elbows
8 burpees to target
8 single arm dumbbell overhead squats

LEVEL III
8 rounds for time:
8 toes to bar
8 burpees to target
8 single arm dumbbell overhead squats

NOTES: Overhead squats should alternate each round, i.e., round 1 is left arm, rounds 2 is right arm. Dumbbell weight is up to you. Target for burpee should be 6 inches (15 cm) or more above reach.

332

LEVEL I
3 rounds for time:
400-meter treadmill run
21 dumbbell swings
12 jumping pullups

LEVEL II
3 rounds for time:
400-meter treadmill run
21 dumbbell swings
12 pullups

LEVEL III
3 rounds for time:
400-meter treadmill run
21 dumbbell swings
12 pullups

NOTES: Adjust dumbbell weight to a level where 21 consecutive reps is possible. Swings should be American style (overhead).

333

LEVEL I
3 rounds for time:
5 flights of stairs (up and down)
10 pushups

LEVEL II
4 rounds for time:
5 flights of stairs (up and down)
15 pushups

LEVEL III
5 rounds for time:
5 flights of stairs (up and down)
20 pushups

NOTE: Use hotel stairs, if available.

334

LEVEL I
3 rounds for time:
:30 dead hang hold
:30 air squats
:30 wall walk hold
:30 pushups

LEVEL II
4 rounds for time:
:30 dead hang hold
:30 air squats
:30 wall handstand hold
:30 pushups

LEVEL III
5 rounds for time:
:30 dead hang hold
:30 air squats
:30 wall handstand hold
:30 pushups

NOTES: At level I, take 30 seconds between exercises. At level II, take 15 seconds between exercises. At level III, transition immediately.

WODs ON THE ROAD

335

LEVEL I
3 rounds for time:
10 dumbbell bench presses
20 lateral bench step overs
30 walking lunges

LEVEL II
4 rounds for time:
10 dumbbell bench presses
20 lateral bench jump overs
30 walking lunges

LEVEL III
5 rounds for time:
10 dumbbell bench presses
20 lateral bench jump overs
30 dumbbell walking lunges

NOTES: Dumbbells can be any weight. At level I, step over bench; At level II and level III, place hands on bench and hop over and back.

336

LEVEL I
8-minute AMRAP:
2 laps freestyle
2 laps overhead dumbbell carry
2 laps breaststroke

LEVEL II
10-minute AMRAP:
2 laps freestyle
2 laps overhead dumbbell carry
2 laps breaststroke

LEVEL III
12-minute AMRAP:
2 laps freestyle
2 laps overhead dumbbell carry
2 laps breaststroke

NOTES: Dumbbell does not need to be heavy. Goal is to keep it dry.

337

LEVEL I
Run 1-mile (1.6 km) on treadmill for time
EMOTM complete 2 burpees

LEVEL II
Run 2-miles (3.2 km) on treadmill for time
EMOTM complete 3 burpees

LEVEL III
Run 3-miles (4.8 km) on treadmill for time
EMOTM complete 3 burpees

NOTES: Buy in each minute with the prescribed number of burpees off of the treadmill and then jump on and run as far as possible in the remaining time. Leaving the treadmill running between rounds is recommended.

338

LEVEL I
For time:
Run a parking garage bottom to top
Every 2 levels perform 10 squats, 10 pushups, 10 lunges

LEVEL II
For time:
Run a parking garage bottom to top
Every level perform 10 squats, 10 pushups, 10 lunges

LEVEL III
For time:
Run a parking garage bottom to top
Every level perform 15 squats, 15 pushups, 15 lunges

NOTE: Maximum height of garage should be 10 floors.

339

LEVEL I
12-minute AMRAP:
1-mile (1.6 km) stationary bike
400-meter treadmill run
20 dumbbell thrusters

LEVEL II
16-minute AMRAP:
1-mile (1.6 km) stationary bike
400-meter treadmill run
20 dumbbell thrusters

LEVEL III
20-minute AMRAP:
1-mile (1.6 km) stationary bike
400-meter treadmill run
20 dumbbell thrusters

NOTES: Dumbbells can be any weight. Begin the workout slowly and try to maintain the same pace throughout.

340

LEVEL I
EMOTM; 10-minutes:
1 pullup
2 burpees
20 single unders

LEVEL II
EMOTM; 15-minutes:
1 muscle up
2 burpees
20 double unders

LEVEL III
EMOTM; 20-minutes:
1 muscle up
2 burpees
30 double unders

NOTES: Complete one round of the prescribed work every minute. If you fail to complete a round in the minute, rest the following minute and then resume the workout.

WODs ON THE ROAD

341

LEVEL I
50 knees to elbows for time
Every broken set complete
5 burpees

LEVEL II
75 toes to bar for time
Every broken set complete
5 burpees

LEVEL III
100 toes to bar for time
Every broken set complete
10 burpees

NOTES: The goal is to complete the prescribed knees to elbows/toes to bar in the fastest time possible. The goal is also to complete it in as few sets as possible. Record time and sets completed.

342

LEVEL I
3 rounds for completion:
:30 treading water
5 poolside muscle ups
10 air squats

LEVEL II
4 rounds for completion:
:30 treading water
8 poolside muscle ups
15 air squats

LEVEL III
5 rounds for completion:
:30 treading water without hands
10 poolside muscle ups
20 air squats

NOTES: At level III, tread water with hands above the surface. Poolside muscle ups should be done from straight arms and head under water.

343

LEVEL I
6-x-400-meter treadmill sprints
:30 plank + 1:30 rest between efforts

LEVEL II
8-x-400-meter treadmill sprints
:45 plank + 1:15 rest between efforts

LEVEL III
10-x-400-meter treadmill sprints
1:00 plank + 1:00 rest between efforts

NOTES: Pace for sprints should be 85 to 90 percent. Planks and rest between sprints should be done next to treadmill.

344

LEVEL I
3 rounds for time:
500-meter row
10 dumbbell bench presses
10 dumbbell front squats

LEVEL II
3 rounds for time:
750-meter row
15 dumbbell bench presses
15 dumbbell front squats

LEVEL III
3 rounds for time:
1000-meter row
20 dumbbell bench presses
20 dumbbell front squats

NOTE: Dumbbells can be any weight.

345

LEVEL I
EMOTM; 10-minutes:
5 ring rows
5 pushups
10 air squats

LEVEL II
EMOTM; 15-minutes:
5 ring rows
5 ring pushups
10 squat jumps

LEVEL III
EMOTM; 20-minutes:
5 ring rows
5 ring pushups
10 squat jumps

NOTES: Ring rows/pushups can be adjusted for difficulty by raising or lowering rings. Jumps don't need to be just high enough to see ground clearance.

346

LEVEL I
3 rounds for completion:
400-meter treadmill run
4 crouched headstand to crow
20 dumbbell push presses

LEVEL II
4 rounds for completion:
400-meter treadmill run
6 full headstand to crow
20 dumbbell push presses

LEVEL III
5 rounds for completion:
400-meter treadmill run
10 full headstand to crow
20 dumbbell push presses

NOTES: All headstands are done with hands on the ground for support. The movement to crow pose should be slow and controlled, bringing the knees down from headstand to balance on the elbows until the head can be raised off the ground. Push press can be done at any weight.

WODs ON THE ROAD

347

LEVEL I
3 rounds for completion:
10 dumbbell split squats
10 dumbbell ground to overheads
10 man makers

LEVEL II
4 rounds for completion:
10 dumbbell split squats
10 dumbbell ground to overheads
10 man makers

LEVEL III
5 rounds for completion:
10 dumbbell split squats
10 dumbbell ground to overheads
10 man makers

NOTES: Dumbbells can be any weight. Split squats should be performed with dumbbells on shoulders. Ground to overheads can be performed in any fashion. Man makers are done from a pushup position, alternating between pushups and dumbbell rows.

348

LEVEL I
For time:
400-meter run
10 dumbbell thrusters
10 burpees
200-meter run
20 dumbbell thrusters
20 burpees
100-meter run
30 dumbbell thrusters
30 burpees

LEVEL II
800-meter run
10 dumbbell thrusters
10 burpees
400-meter run
20 dumbbell thrusters
20 burpees
200-meter run
30 dumbbell thrusters
30 burpees

LEVEL III
1-mile (1.6 km) run
10 dumbbell thrusters
10 burpees
800-meter run
20 dumbbell thrusters
20 burpees
400-meter run
30 dumbbell thrusters
30 burpees

NOTE: Dumbbells can be any weight.

349

LEVEL I
21-15-9 for time:
Pushups
Ring rows
Air squats

LEVEL II
21-15-9 for time:
Ring dips
Ring rows
Deck squats

LEVEL III
21-18-15-9-6 for time:
Ring dips
Ring rows
Deck squats

NOTE: At level I and level II, you may use hands to assist deck squats.

350

LEVEL I
EMOTM; 10-minutes:
5 alternating single arm dumbbell swings
5 alternating single arm dumbbell thrusters

LEVEL II
EMOTM; 15-minutes:
5 alternating single arm dumbbell swings
5 alternating single arm dumbbell thrusters

LEVEL III
EMOTM; 20-minutes:
5 alternating single arm dumbbell swings
5 alternating single arm dumbbell thrusters

NOTES: Dumbbell swings should be Russian style (eye level) and can be any weight. Thrusters should change hands when the dumbbell is at chest level.

351

LEVEL I
For time:
400-meter uphill treadmill walk (15 degree incline)
50 jumping pullups
100 pushups
150 air squats
400-meter uphill treadmill walk (15 degree incline)

LEVEL II
For time:
600-meter uphill treadmill walk (15 degree incline)
75 pullups
150 pushups
200 air squats
600-meter uphill treadmill walk (15 degree incline)

LEVEL III
For time:
800-meter uphill treadmill walk (15 degree incline)
100 pullups
200 pushups
300 air squats
800-meter uphill treadmill walk (15 degree incline)

NOTES: You determine how fast to walk the hill. Pullups, pushups, and air squats can be divided up however necessary in order to finish the total set.

352

LEVEL I
10-minute AMRAP:
3 burpees
3 jumping pullups
6 burpees
6 jumping pullups
9 burpees
9 jumping pullups
(and so forth)

LEVEL II
10-minute AMRAP:
3 burpees
3 pullups
6 burpees
6 pullups
9 burpees
9 pullups
(and so forth)

LEVEL III
10-minute AMRAP:
3 burpees
3 pullups
6 burpees
6 pullups
9 burpees
9 pullups
(and so forth)

NOTE: You climb the repetition ladder as high as you can in 10 minutes.

353

LEVEL I
2 rounds for time using 2 flights of stairs:
Two-foot jump up
Jog down
Right foot step up
10 pushups
Jog down
Left foot step up
Jog down
Run up
10 pushups
Jog down

LEVEL II
3 rounds for time using 2 flights of stairs:
Two-foot jump up
Jog down
Right foot jump up
Bear crawl down
Left foot jump up
Jog down
Run up
Bear crawl down

LEVEL III
5 rounds for time using 2 flights of stairs:
Two-foot jump up
Jog down
Right foot jump up
Bear crawl down
Left foot jump up
Jog down
Run up
Bear crawl down

NOTES: All jumping and crawling movements should be done with great care and precision. Any staircase will work; use gloves if outside.

354

LEVEL I
8-minute AMRAP:
5 dumbbell strict presses
5 dumbbell push presses
5 dumbbell push jerks
400-meter treadmill run

LEVEL II
10-minute AMRAP:
5 dumbbell strict presses
5 dumbbell push presses
5 dumbbell push jerks
400-meter treadmill run

LEVEL III
12-minute AMRAP:
5 dumbbell strict presses
5 dumbbell push presses
5 dumbbell push jerks
400-meter treadmill run

NOTES: Dumbbell weights should be chosen to complete 5 strict presses with difficulty. Attempt to complete the lifting portions unbroken.

355

LEVEL I
3 rounds for time:
500-meter row
20 dumbbell ground to overheads
15 knees to elbows
10 pushups

LEVEL II
3 rounds for time:
500-meter row
20 dumbbell ground to overheads
15 toes to bar
10 piked pushups

LEVEL III
3 rounds for time:
500-meter row
30 dumbbell ground to overheads
20 toes to bar
10 handstand pushups

NOTES: Dumbbells can be any weight and may move from ground to overhead in any fashion while maintaining good technique and back support.

356

LEVEL I
21-15-9 for time:
Dumbbell deadlifts
Step ups

LEVEL II
21-15-9 for time:
Dumbbell deadlifts
Box jumps

LEVEL III
21-18-15-9-6 for time:
Dumbbell deadlifts
Box jumps

NOTES: Dumbbells should be heavy to simulate the intensity of a barbell deadlift. Box jumps can be done on a bench or ledge.

357

LEVEL I
1-mile (1.6 km) uphill object carry (5 degree incline)

LEVEL II
1-mile (1.6 km) uphill object carry (10 degree incline)

LEVEL III
1-mile (1.6 km) uphill object carry (15 degree incline)

NOTES: Object can be a dumbbell, medicine ball, etc. Can be carried in any fashion.

358

LEVEL I
Perform an additional dumbbell hang squat clean thruster EMOTM until failure to complete (20 pounds [9 kg]/10 pounds [4.5 kg])
1 in minute 1
2 in minute 2
3 in minute 3
(and so forth)

LEVEL II
Perform an additional dumbbell hang squat clean thruster EMOTM until failure to complete (30 pounds [13.5 kg]/15 pounds [7 kg])
1 in minute 1
2 in minute 2
3 in minute 3
(and so forth)

LEVEL III
Perform an additional dumbbell hang squat clean thruster EMOTM until failure to complete (40 pounds [18 kg]/25 pounds [[11.5 kg])
1 in minute 1
2 in minute 2
3 in minute 3
(and so forth)

NOTES: Dumbbells must be cleaned to the shoulders as the athlete goes into a front squat, then pressed overhead as the athlete stands up.

359

LEVEL I
3 rounds for completion:
10 situps
10 good mornings
10 lunges
50 single unders

LEVEL II
4 rounds for completion:
10 weighted situps
10 weighted good mornings
10 weighted lunges
30 double unders

LEVEL III
5 rounds for completion:
10 weighted situps
10 weighted good mornings
10 weighted lunges
50 double unders

NOTES: Dumbbells or medicine balls can be used to weight all exercises. Weight should not exceed 20 pounds (9 kg).

360

LEVEL I

For time:
Carry-10 pound (4.5 kg) dumbbells up 5 flights of stairs
Carry-20 pound (9 kg) dumbbells up 5 flights of stairs
Carry-30 pound (13.5 kg) dumbbells up 5 flights of stairs
Complete 30 burpees
Carry-30 pound (13.5 kg) dumbbells down 5 flights
Carry-20 pound (9 kg) dumbbells down 5 flights
Carry-10 pound (4.5 kg) dumbbells down 5 flights

LEVEL II

For time:
Carry-15 pound (7 kg) dumbbells up 5 flights of stairs
Carry-25 pound (11.5 kg) dumbbells up 5 flights of stairs
Carry-35 pound (16 kg) dumbbells up 5 flights of stairs
Complete 40 burpees
Carry-35 pound (16 kg) dumbbells down 5 flights
Carry-25 pound (11.5 kg) dumbbells down 5 flights
Carry-15 pound (7 kg) dumbbells down 5 flights

LEVEL III

For time:
Carry-20 pound (9 kg) dumbbells up 5 flights of stairs
Carry-30 pound (13.5 kg) dumbbells up 5 flights of stairs
Carry-40 pound (18 kg) dumbbells up 5 flights of stairs
Complete 50 burpees
Carry-40 pound (18 kg) dumbbells down 5 flights
Carry-30 pound (13.5 kg) dumbbells down 5 flights
Carry-20 pound (9 kg) dumbbells down 5 flights

NOTES: Use hotel stairs if available. If no stairs, use treadmill. Dumbbells can be carried in any fashion.

363

LEVEL I

10-minute AMRAP:
¼-mile (400 m) stationary bike sprint
10 hollow rocks
10 dumbbell deadlifts
10 dumbbell floor presses

LEVEL II

15-minute AMRAP:
¼-mile (400 m) stationary bike sprint
10 knees to elbows
10 dumbbell deadlifts
10 dumbbell floor presses

LEVEL III

20-minute AMRAP:
½-mile (800 m) stationary bike sprint
10 toes to bar
10 dumbbell deadlifts
10 dumbbell floor presses

NOTES: Dumbbells can be any weight. Floor presses should be controlled so that both elbows contact the floor at the same time before pressing out.

WODs ON THE ROAD

362

LEVEL I
100 dumbbell hang cleans for time
EMOTM complete 5 push presses

LEVEL II
100 dumbbell hang cleans for time
EMOTM complete 5 push presses

LEVEL III
100 dumbbell hang cleans for time
EMOTM complete 5 push presses

NOTES: Dumbbells should be scaled to a weight where 10 consecutive repetitions are possible. Goal is to finish in less than 10 minutes.

363

LEVEL I
30-20-10 for time:
Single dumbbell swings
Pushups

LEVEL II
30-20-10 for time:
Double dumbbell swings
Bar dips

LEVEL III
30-20-10 for time:
Double dumbbell swings
Ring dips

NOTES: Dumbbells can be any weight. Swings should be American style (overhead) and the dumbbells should be kept next to one another. At level I, swing a single dumbbell using both hands.

364

LEVEL I
Complete maximum repetitions in 1-minute for each of the following exercises:
Pushups
Pullups
Situps
Squats
Toes to bar
Ring dips
Lunges

LEVEL II
Complete maximum repetitions in 1-minute for each of the following exercises:
Pushups
Pullups

Situps
Squats
Toes to bar
Ring dips
Lunges

LEVEL III

Complete maximum unbroken repetitions in 1-minute for each of the following exercises:

Pushups
Pullups
Situps
Squats
Toes to bar
Ring dips
Lunges

NOTES: Rest as long as needed between exercises, give yourself only 1 minute to complete the reps for each. Only consecutive reps will count for level III.

365

LEVEL I

10-minute AMRAP:
30 unbroken single unders
20 dumbbell shoulder to overheads
10 burpees over box

LEVEL II

15-minute AMRAP:
30 double unders
20 dumbbell shoulder to overheads
10 burpees over box

LEVEL III

20-minute AMRAP:
30 unbroken double unders
20 dumbbell shoulder to overheads
10 burpees over box

NOTES: Dumbbells can be any weight. Benches or ledges can be used for burpees over box. Stepping up and over is allowed for level I, but at level II and level III jump onto the box must be two footed before stepping down on the other side.

ABOUT THE AUTHOR

Blair Morrison played football and studied history at Princeton University before entering the fitness industry, in 2005. He has competed in CrossFit at the highest level, qualifying for the 2009, 2010, and 2011 games as an individual competitor, finishing seventh, twenty-second, and fifth, respectively. He opened CrossFit Anywhere in 2011 and currently runs guided fitness-adventure tours around the world.

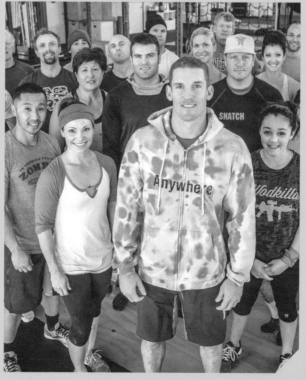

He is a product of northern California and its unlimited supply of rivers, lakes, open spaces, and sun. As an athlete in high school and in college, he faced the challenge of being too small, too weak, and too slow to keep up with his peers. He was drawn to the pain and simplicity of training because it offered a way to change this. Following his undergraduate degree, he spent three years personal training at Balance Gym in Washington, D.C. Here, he was exposed to almost everything the fitness world had to offer: bodybuilding, Pilates, rehab, yoga, you name it. In 2009, he left the United States to study European History at Universiteit Leiden, Sorbonne, and Oxford. During this time, he was forced to reimagine what fitness could be for an individual living without the standard resources of a gym. These experiences have taught him to pursue the physical challenges our bodies were built to face and appreciate the mental fortitude that comes from the ability to overcome them.

INDEX